ULTIMATE

FITNESS

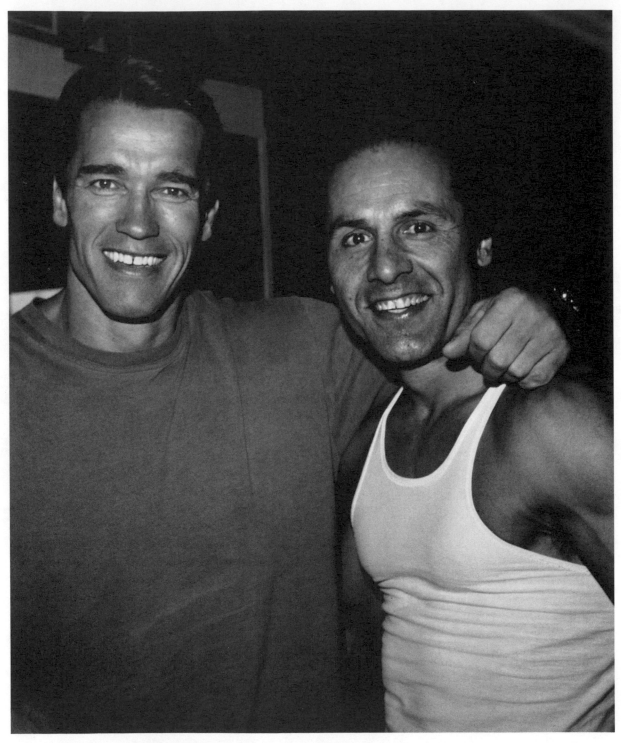

Two champions having a good time after a workout *(Photo by Art Zeller)*

ULTIMATE FITNESS

DAVID LUNA

President, Fitness Professionals of America
Santa Monica, California

Illustrated with 110 Photographs
by John Balik

ROUNDTABLE PUBLISHING, INC.
Santa Monica California

ROUNDTABLE PUBLISHING, INC.
933 Pico Boulevard
Santa Monica, CA 90405

First Printing, 1989

Library of Congress Catalog Card Number—88-61234

ISBN—0-915677-38-5

PRINTED IN THE UNITED STATES OF AMERICA

This book is dedicated to my grandmother, Nelly.

ACKNOWLEDGMENTS

I wish to thank the following people for their assistance, support, and influence in the creation of this book:

My beautiful wife, Kathy, and our lovely daughter, Jennifer;

My wonderful mom;

Harold Bailey, M.D., F.A.C.S., cardiologist;

John Balik, one of the world's best photographers;

Lorrie Chappas, RPT, Los Angeles;

Larry Dreschler, Pharm. D., Hendricks Pharmacy, Claremont, CA;

Peter Dyck, M.D., P.A.C.S., St. Vincente Medical Center, Los Angeles;

V. Reggie Edgerton, Ph.D, Chairman and professor of kinesiology, UCLA;

George Elmstrom, O.D., American Optometric Association;

Mary Felando, M.S., R.D., clinical dietician;

Sondra Feldmen, RN, and behavioral modification specialist, St. John's Hospital, Santa Monica, CA;

Gerald Gardner, Ph.D, emeritus professor of kinesiology, UCLA;

James Gernert, M.D., F.A.C.S., Chief of Staff, Hollywood Presbyterian Hospital, Los Angeles;

Joe Gold, owner of World Gym, Venice, CA;

Ida Jaqua, R.D., my first nutrition professor, Los Angeles;

James Kenney, Ph.D., R.D., Pritikin Longevity Center, Santa Monica;

Arnold Kline, RPT, Los Angeles;

Joon Koh, M.D., F.A.C.S., Queen of Angels Medical Center, Los Angeles;

Bruce Lee and Dan Inosanto, my respects to two great martial artists;

Robin McKenzie, back specialist, M.N.Z.S.P., M.N.Z.M.T.A., New Zealand;

Monica Leigh Perdue for a well done modeling assignment;

Nathan Pritikin, founder of the Longevity Center, Santa Monica;

Bernie Quintero, Director of Corporate Development, Queen of Angels Medical Center, Los Angeles;

Michael Schiffman, M.D., American Academy of Orthopedic Surgeons, Centinela Hospital, Los Angeles;

Barbara Stone, RPT, South Bay Spine Center, Torrance, CA;

Henry Siegel and Karen Voight,

Roz Sullivan, for giving me my first job at the Beverly Hills Health Club;

Arnold Schwarzenegger;

Sylvester Stallone;

Leonard Tyminski, M.D., Queen of Angels Medical Center, Los Angeles;

Ursula Weatherton, M.S., R.D., clinical dietician, Riverside Community Hospital, Riverside, CA;

Joel Yager, M.D., Program Director, Eating Disorder Clinic, UCLA Neuropsychiatric Institute, Los Angeles;

Marcy Clements, Norma Lynn Cutler, Brenda Eagerton, Lee Tescher and Bernie Zavidowski for editorial assistance;

Isgo Lepejian, for printing most of the black and white photographs;

And last, but not least, my students, clients, co-workers and friends.

CONTENTS

We squander health
In search of wealth;
We scheme and toil and save;
Then squander wealth
In search of health
And all we get's a grave.
We live and boast of what we own;
We die and only get a stone.

Anonymous

ULTIMATE FITNESS

Introduction

MOTIVATION

Some men are bigger, faster, stronger, and smarter than others—but not a single man has a corner on dreams, desire, or ambition.

—Duffy Daugherty

Last year, I attended a three-day seminar on sports psychology given by Dr. Gregory Raiport, sports psychologist for the 1976 Soviet Olympic team. There, I learned something about motivation that I had been doing for years, but had not previously analyzed scientifically.

Dr. Raiport's seminar centered around auto-conditioning training, which involves the ability of the subject to learn to generate peak performance at will. We all have this innate ability. However, most of us do not know how to utilize it toward achieving success. Dr. Raiport defined a successful person as one who: (1) likes, loves, or enjoys what he or she does; (2) is able to focus his or her attention; (3) has the courage to explore new things; (4) believes that he or she is worthy or deserving of success; (5) is able to visualize or use imagery.

Every one of you reading this has had difficulty with motivation at one time or another. But what is motivation and how does one obtain it? Paul Young, in his book *Motivation and Emotion,* defines it as the "process of arousing action, sustaining the activity in progress, and regulating the pattern of activity." Dr. Raiport defines motivation as an "elevation of the level of concern toward a specific goal." In general, motivation means "to move or to activate." As

president of Fitness Professionals of America, I know my company is aware that motivation affects the success of the hundreds of people with whom we work.

A study by Dr. Allen Roberts at Scripps Clinic in La Jolla found the following individuals to have a high dropout rate:

1. Smokers
2. Overweight people
3. Type A personalities (irritable, agressive etc.)
4. Those with poor credit ratings
5. Injury-prone individuals
6. Those on high-intensity exercise
7. Those who do not set goals
8. Those who fail to achieve goals
9. Those with spouses who do not support their exercise programs
10. Those who exercise alone
11. Those with increased coronary risk factors
12. Those with an excessive amount of unstructured leisure time

Beyond Dr. Roberts' study, there are other important factors to consider. One must remember that one's perception of life becomes

1

one's reality. So often people say to me, "I just don't seem to have the discipline." I normally ask, "Why?" And the response is, "I don't know. I just don't!" If you say to yourself, "I can't," do you know why you will not succeed? You just said it, "I can't!"

Secondly, personal as well as professional achievements are based on adherence. Dr. James Rippe, director of the exercise physiology laboratory at the University of Massachusetts Medical School, says, "of every two people who start an exercise program, one drops out within six months." That's why the ten most important words in the English language are: "IF IT IS TO BE, IT IS UP TO ME!"

The following are a few suggestions for developing and maintaining motivation:

1. Use positive reinforcement. It is the most potent of all strategies. "Motivation is highly related to the principle of effect, *i.e.,* people are more likely to have high motivation when they are succeeding than otherwise."[1]
2. Dress the part. It's the external preparation. Also, wear something that you look and feel good in and that allows mobility.
3. Exercise to music. With music, exercise is perceived as being less stressful and more enjoyable.
4. Surround yourself with people who think the same as you do—preferably people who are into health, fitness, and growth. If you associate with people who are not supportive or who do not actively engage in fitness, you are less likely to succeed.
5. Exercise with a friend or in a group situation rather than alone. Exercise done in groups is generally more successful.
6. Hire a competent private trainer to work with you.
7. Define your goals and be clear about how you plan to attain them. Clarity of vision is a powerful tool.
8. Use the variety conditioning concept. In other words, integrate a wide variety of activities that you enjoy. Also, place emphasis on your cardiovascular system, strength, flexibility, and coordination.
9. Schedule a time for your fitness activities or exercise program. If you leave it to chance, it will never happen. Schedule it into your calendar, just as you would all your other appointments. Nathan Pritikin once said, "In so far as exercise is concerned, there is no convenient time to exercise. You have to make the time."
10. Employ self-monitoring (record keeping). Self-monitoring enhances compliance, particularly when supplemented with positive reinforcement. Note frequency of workouts, body weight, and if desired, distance walked, run, or cycled. Repetitions and levels of weights may be noted weekly if desired. Winners keep records!
11. Employ self-contracting. Write down exactly what you choose to do, date and sign it. The following is an example of self-contracting:

> I, John Doe, hereby make this agreement with myself, that I will exercise for thirty minutes three times per week. I also agree that I will lose a minimum of one pound per week and preferably no more than two pounds per week until I reach my ideal bodyweight of 160 pounds. I willfully make this agreement.
>
> John Doe
> May 15, 1989

Make self-contracting goals realistic and attainable. Contract (if you wish) with a close friend or clinician. Forget about New Year's resolutions. They're a waste of time!
12. Focus on the benefits of exercise. If you see that your weight is dropping, endurance and strength are increasing, body fat is decreasing, and blood pressure is improving—you have some strong motivating forces working in your favor. Use them to your advantage.
13. Take advantage of all the new high-tech

equipment that is out on the market. Computer-programmed exercise equipment with instant visual feedback and user programmability increases people's likelihood of adhering to exercise.

14. "One of the best methods of motivating an athlete is to raise his or her level of aspiration, that is, the level of skill he or she thinks can be achieved. This should be accomplished gradually, from a lower level of aspiration to a higher but realistic level."[2]

15. Use imagery and visualization. These are powerful techniques. Visualize yourself being where you would like to be, what you would like to be doing, or what you would like to look like. If you want to be thin, you have to conceptualize yourself being thin. Create a mental photo of exactly what you want, then take the necessary steps to make it a reality.

Whenever I run, for example, I try to imitate the speed and grace of a cheetah. I allow myself to blend with the wind. When I stair train (running up and down stairs), I imagine that someone is behind me, pushing me up the stairs.

During most of the eighties, I had a ten-thousand-dollar fitness challenge to any man in the world who could follow me through a ninety-minute workout. I had extended the challenge to both the Soviet Union and the People's Republic of China. I wanted to compete against their top athletes. I recall that, during my training, I always imagined there was a Russian or a Chinese athlete right behind me doing everything that I was doing. This forced me to train harder, for I was determined not to allow anyone to follow me through a workout.

Karate expert Chuck Norris, during his tournament years, would first fight his opponents mentally, secondly, defeat them mentally, and thirdly, defeat them physically.

Sometimes, when I'm working with clients, I have them imagine their body fat dripping off their hips, thighs, and midsection and have them see and feel their bodies getting stronger as they're working out. I frequently visualize my body fat eroding as I'm running and rope jumping along the ocean.

The important thing is to use your imagination to visually create and mold what you want, then to go out and get it. Don't be like the man at the bottom of the well who looks up at the sky and thinks that the only part of the sky he sees is all that there is to heaven. Whatever you can conceive, you can achieve!

16. Allow your motivation to evolve from the things that are most important in your life: (a) your family; (b) your health; (c) your job; (d) your religious beliefs.

In conclusion, I want to say that there is no single way to motivate. Consideration of each individual's interests, aspirations, attitudes, abilities, and anxiety level is needed to determine the most effective means of inspiration. Most of the great athletes, artists, musicians, businessmen and women, and world leaders have been highly motivated people. But the common denominator has been that they knew where they were going, knew what they wanted, and aligned themselves with that goal in mind. Motivation has nothing to do with luck. It lies within yourself, waiting to be activated and directed. So activate yourself and move powerfully with boldness and clearness of vision!

INTRODUCTION NOTES

[1] Sherill, Claudine, *Adapted Physical Education and Recreation* (Dubuque, Iowa: William C. Brown Co., 1981), p. 102.

[2] *Fundamentals of Athletic Training,* National Athletic Trainers Association and the American Medical Association (Chicago, Illinois, 1975), p. 40.

Part I

THE LUNA
EXERCISE
PROGRAM

Chapter 1

THE LUNA METHOD

Never be like the man at the bottom of the well who looks up at the sky
and thinks the only part of the sky he sees is all that there is to heaven.

The Luna Method is a new and unique approach to physical conditioning that women and men alike will find enjoyable, adaptable, and effective. Not another fad, the Luna Method is a product of 17 years of development and testing in association with (1) Fitness Professionals of America, Santa Monica, CA; (2) The Claremont Club in Claremont, CA; (3) Voight Fitness and Dance Center, Los Angeles; (4) Queen of Angels Medical Center, Los Angeles; (5) Midway Hospital Medical Center, Los Angeles; and (6) The Beverly Hills Country Club.

The Luna Method is involved with growth and the development of human potential. In other words, being better today than you were yesterday.

The Luna Method will provide you with a step-by-step approach to the "look" of the nineties—a healthy, well-proportioned, symmetrical, lean look.

The Luna Method starts with five basic training components:

1. Flexibility
2. Endurance
3. Strength
4. Balance and coordination
5. Definition

All five will be equally developed, unless of course, there are some areas that require more time and attention than others. Restricting your program to one or two of these areas is self-limiting.

The Luna Method also introduces the following concepts:

MULTIFUNCTIONAL EXERCISE

Multifunctional exercise is a training concept that I developed in the early 1980s. It is based on working as many different body parts as possible during one exercise. The only stipulation with multifunctional exercise is that you isolate the primary muscle being worked. If you are unable to do this, this conditioning concept loses its efficacy, because of the tendency to "cheat" or use inertia—the force generated by swinging.

The advantages of multifunctional exercises are obvious: (a) when applied properly, you are able to work two or three different body parts simultaneously; (b) you accomplish much more during your allotted exercise time. Multifunctional exercise is perfect for the man or woman who has very little time or who chooses to spend very little time in the gym.

If you are at a beginning level, apply this concept slowly, gradually, and progressively as tolerated. Maintaining control and using sound biomechanic techniques are of utmost importance. It takes a lot more energy, but the results are worth it. Apply this training concept within reason, preferably under the guidance of a competent private trainer or fitness consultant.

The following are a few examples of multi-functional exercises:

Quarter Sit-ups with Alternate Elbow to Knee Combination

Quarter sit-ups are an upper abdominal exercise, but by using the lower extremities and alternating right elbow to left knee, and vice versa, you can simultaneously work the lower abdominals, obliques, hip flexors, anterior thighs, and the shin muscles, by keeping your feet pointed towards you. (See Figure 1-1.)

Side Leg Raises Standing on the Ball of Weightbearing Foot

Side leg raises is an exercise that primarily works the outer thighs. By standing on the ball of the foot, you can also work the calf; and by keeping the arm extended out, you are able to tone the shoulder. (See Figure 1-2.)

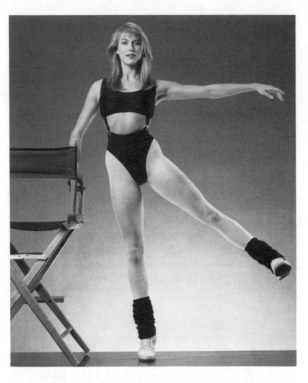

Figure 1-2. Side Leg Raises Standing on the Ball of Weightbearing Foot.

Running and Rope Jumping Simultaneously

(See Figure 1-3.)

Figure 1-1. Quarter Sit-ups with Alternate Elbow to Knee Combination.

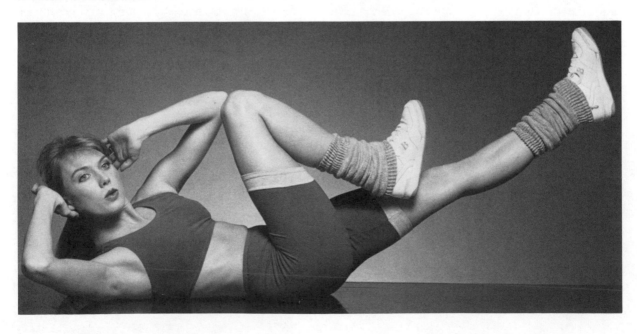

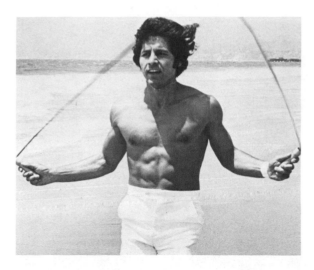

Figure 1-3. Running and Rope-Jumping Simultaneously. *(Photo by Erik Stern.)*

Continuous Movement

Continuous movement is an optional training technique for someone at an advanced level of training only. It is not recommended for anyone at a beginning level. It is a type of circuit training that requires going from one exercise to another with either very little rest or no rest at all. The "in-between exercises" may consist of jogging in place, calisthenics, abdominal exercises, rowing, Stairmaster, lunges, knee-bends, rope-jumping, or stationary cycling. Once you start training, you don't stop until you're finished. Obviously if you need to take a breather, stop, check your pulse, and then continue when you're ready. Pace yourself and make sure all training is well tolerated.

There are several reasons for the continuous movement:

1. Constant movement enables you to keep your pulse rate elevated throughout your workout, thereby increasing stamina and caloric expenditure and decreasing body fat.
2. The mind remains more focused and concentrated on the workout.
3. You are able to maintain a more constant rhythm and flow with your training.
4. Body temperature remains elevated throughout the workout.

5. Mild exercise, such as jogging, between the heavier bursts of activity may be advantageous, since the elimination of lactic acid is faster than at complete rest.[1] Lactic acid is the substance that is formed in the muscles during activity by the breakdown of glycogen (reserve fuel). It is also thought to be one of the substances that causes muscle soreness.
6. If working out with weights, you are able to concentrate on both strength and endurance at the same time by combining the weight training with the aerobics. This works out very well for people who don't have a lot of time to exercise.

Those at beginning and intermediate levels should not attempt to maintain continuous movement. Allow instead for rest periods in between exercises. Gradually start out with whatever you can do, and progressively increase from there. *Never* double repetitions, weight, mileage, intensity, duration, or frequency unless you want to have a short athletic career. I've seen too many people get caught up in the "too much, too soon syndrome" and end up with knee and back problems, hernias, "tennis elbow," chest pain, heart attacks, "shin splints," torn rotator cuffs, etc. All training should be done as tolerated. Get a physical check-up and exercise within your doctor's recommendations. Refer to Table III-1 to determine your appropriate training intensity.

Table I-1 SEQUENCE TRAINING	
Quadriceps	Chest
Hamstrings	Biceps
Calves	Shoulders
Inner thighs	Back
Outer thighs	Lower abdominals
Buttocks	Triceps
Thighs	Upper abdominals

Heavy/Light Workouts

The Luna Method consists of training heavy one day and light the next. Going all-out every day is self-defeating. It not only increases the risk of injury, but could cause "burn out" as well. Therefore, vary your workouts, as well as the level of intensity. Your "light" workouts may consist of stretching, a short run, a brisk walk, swimming, or cycling. The "heavy" workouts may consist of weight training, a long or fast-paced run, or a competitive game of tennis or racquetball. The only real difference between a "heavy" and a "light" workout is the level of intensity, resistance, and duration.

The suggested activities listed as "light" workouts can very easily be upgraded to "heavy" by merely increasing the intensity, resistance, duration, or degree of difficulty. Train at a level that you feel is right for you and intermittently check your pulse.

SOUND BIOMECHANICS— FORM AND TECHNIQUE

Good biomechanics, form and technique, are crucial to any training program. They provide a solid foundation from which to grow. Professionals have good form, good technique, and sound biomechanics. They are what separates professionals from amateurs. Without these three elements, the probability of injury increases significantly and results are often "hit and miss." The bottom line is: If you're going to train, do it right!

Pictured here are examples of good and bad biomechanics, form, and technique.

Inertia Elimination

The use of inertia (also known as "cheating") in training is an error that is observed not only in beginners but with advanced athletes as well.

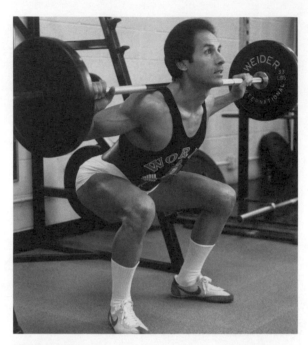

Figure 1-4. Proper Method of Executing a 90 degree Knee Bend.

Figure 1-5. Knee Hyperflexion. Overstresses knees and ankles.

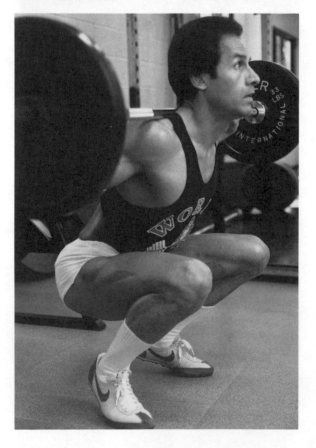

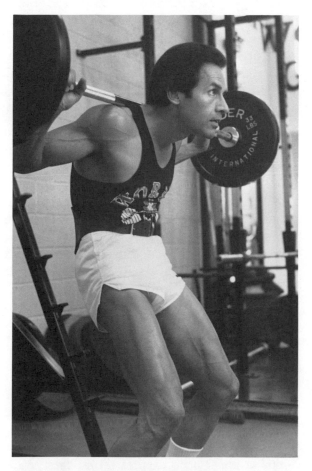

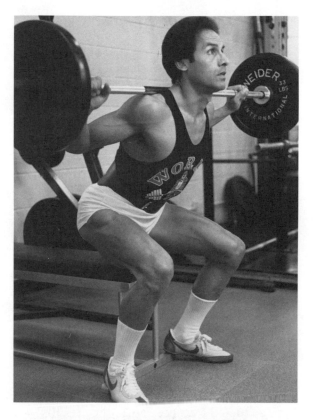

Figure 1-8. Potential Back Compression.

Figure 1-6. Potential Back Strain.

Figure 1-7. Potential Back Strain.

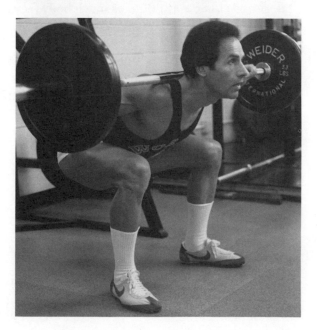

Inertia elimination is the absence of "momentum" to assist in lifting or lowering a weight. Inertia occurs primarily with the use of free weights and pulleys, but can also be done using Nautilus or similar equipment. Inertia is frequently observed in men doing standing dumbbell or barbell curls and in women doing rear leg lifts.

The most effective ways to eliminate inertia are: (a) slow down and work in a more controlled manner; (b) use negative resistance; (c) decrease the weight or resistance.

Negative Resistance

Negative resistance is a training concept that not only emphasizes the lifting of a weight, but the lowering of a weight as well. It's based on the 2-4-1 concept—that is, lift the weight on a quick count of 2, hold the weight stationary for a count of 1, and slowly lower or return the weight to the starting position of the exercise for a count of 4.

Even though negative resistance is difficult to perform, the one thing I like about it is that you're always in control of the weight, instead of the weight controlling you. There's nothing jerky or staccato about it.

One final word. Negative resistance is generally used by athletes and body builders at an advanced level; however, if the weight is light, it can be used by those at an intermediate level, so long as there are no medical restrictions.

Recovery Phase Elimination (RPE)

The RPE concept is simply the elimination of the rest or recovery phase during an exercise. The whole point to RPE is to keep a muscle or group of muscles in a constant state of contraction until the completion of the exercise. Rest at the end of each set, not after each repetition. Most people rest for a fraction of a second after each repetition. The result is a series of muscle contractions followed by relaxation during a set or exercise. In and of itself, it's okay, but limited. Using the RPE concept, the results are significantly greater. Muscle tone and strength are enhanced as a result of constant contractions. You also improve at a much faster rate.

When most people perform sit-ups, for example, they rest the abdominals after each repetition rather than at the end of the set. If you rest the head and shoulders when you return to the starting position, what happens to the abdominals? That's right, they rest too. If you keep the abs contracted, keeping the head and shoulders elevated, avoiding the recovery phase, your workouts will take on a whole new

dimension. If you can only do ten sit-ups without recovery, that's fine. Gradually and progressively work up from there. It's a powerful and effective way to train. Pictured here are two examples of sit-ups with recovery and sit-ups without recovery.

The recovery phase elimination concept also applies to weight training. When the weight is returned to its starting position, allow it to quickly touch or almost touch the other weights on the stack, but not to rest. This applies to equipment such as Universal, Paramount, Nautilus, Marcy, Icarion, and Eagle. The same concept applies to free weights. Keep the muscles involved in a constant state of contraction. If you're a beginner, work at a level that is well tolerated. Start out with a few repetitions and gradually work up.

Sequence Training and Large Muscle Fiber Recruitment

Sequence training is a conditioning concept that is based on working the body's largest muscles (legs) and alternating or super-setting it with an upper-body exercise (arms, chest, back, shoulders, or abdominals). The rationale behind sequence training and large muscle fiber recruitment is threefold: (1) Burn as many calories as possible. (2) Burn as much body fat as possible. (3) Make maximum use of your training time.

The effectiveness of sequence training lies in the alternating of upper and lower extremities. For example, if you're working legs, the next area

Figure 1-9. Incorrect.

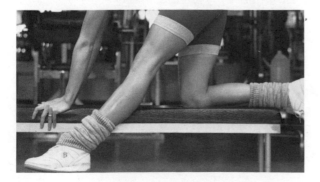

Figure 1-10. Incorrect.

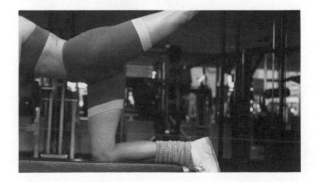

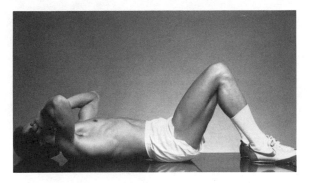

Figure 1-11. Sit-ups with Recovery.

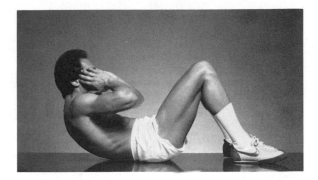

Figure 1-12. Sit-ups without Recovery.

you train is one that is totally unrelated, such as the chest. You then return to legs. Another advantage is that, instead of having to sit around and wait for the area that you just worked to recover, sequence training enables you to immediately move on to another area. The workout is efficient, intense, focused, and concentrated. An example of sequence training can be seen in Tables I-1 and I-2.

Proper Breathing

This one's easy. Breathing procedure while exercising is to exhale on the effort. For example, if you're doing sit-ups, exhale on the way up, inhale on the way down. If you're bench pressing, exhale as you press the barbell up, inhale as you lower the barbell. If you're not sure where to exhale or inhale, evaluate the exercise to determine where you have the greatest amount of effort or exertion. Whatever you do, don't hold your breath. Remember EE: Exhale on Effort.

Mental Focus and Concentration

Mental focus and concentration is one of the more important aspects of the Luna Method. It's a very cerebral and intense type of training. This type of training is not for everyone. It is suited more for someone at an intermediate or advanced level of training. If you want to make significant progress with your workouts, focus totally on the exercise or activity at hand. If you want to have

Table I-2 SEQUENCE TRAINING			
Exercise	*Sets*	*Reps*	*Weight*
90 degree squats—Bench press	2	12	Moderate
Leg curls—Bicep curls	2	12	"
Calf raises—Military press	2	12	"
Outer thigh—Supine bent knees to chest*	2	12	"
Inner thigh—Lat pulldowns	2	12	"
Rear leg raises—Tricep pressdown	2	12	"
Seated leg press—Quarter sit-ups*	2	12	"

* Repetitions for non-weight bearing exercises can be greater than 12 repetitions. They should be as tolerated.

the functional capacity to generate peak performance at will, use mental focus and concentration. The mind should not be on family, business, or financial problems, or social or political events.

Uninvolved, unemotional, and unmotivated exercise is what I refer to as "mechanical training" or "going through the motions." This is the pattern most people fall into. The reasons for exercising are generally vague and void of direction and emotional content. The process is more of a laborious chore for most people. The bottom line is that, from a fitness perspective, "mechanical training" is limited. There is so much more that could be derived with mental focus and concentration.

So the obvious question is, "How do I involve the mind?" You involve the mind or mental focus and concentration the same way that you would when you are being interviewed by someone from the IRS, or when you see a great looking woman or man. Other examples of focus and concentration are when a dog is about to bite you or when you're watching a tie game with thirty seconds on the clock. They all get your attention. You're mentally alert, focused and concentrated. The mind can think of many different things but can only focus on one thought at a time.

The most important quality that successful people have is their ability to control their attention. John F. Kennedy and Ronald Reagan did this very effectively. Actress Meryl Streep does it very well on the screen. Martial artist Bruce Lee was a master at focusing his attention and energy. On many occasions, Arnold Schwarzenegger, Lou Ferrigno, and I work out at the same time at World Gym in Venice, California. The one common denominator that all three of us have (other than wanting to get the best possible workout) is that our attention is totally focused on the task at hand. I have to admit, when I train, I become oblivious to everything around me. It's a form of dis-association with my immediate environment. I become more assertive, emotionally aroused, and aggressive, but in a controlled way. If I want quality workouts and the ability to generate peak performance at will, I must be mentally focused.

When I go in to train, I train. I'm not there to socialize. If I do socialize, it is always after I'm finished.

This has been one of the keys in setting world, American, and personal records. Activate your mental powers and work in conjunction with, not apart from, your mind. You will move forward powerfully, boldly, and convincingly.

VARIETY CONDITIONING

The Luna Method introduces a new way of training called "variety conditioning." I started experimenting with variety conditioning during the early seventies. It is, without a doubt, one of the most important and successful training techniques I've developed. Simply put, variety conditioning is a form of exercise that integrates many training modalities or activities into an exercise program. The nucleus of variety conditioning is the prescribed exercise program, or any similar program that addresses itself to improving problem areas, or potentially harmful conditions such as a poor cardiovascular system, "thunder thighs," "fanny fallout," "spare tires," flabby midsection, poor flexibility, etc. The peripheral activities, which may comprise part of the prescribed exercise program, could consist of some of the following choices:

1. Cycling
2. Aquatic exercises
3. Low-impact aerobics
4. Tennis
5. Jogging
6. Racquetball
7. Hiking
8. Weight training

The Variety Conditioning Concept is set up according to each individual's preferences. It doesn't have to be limited to just one specific activity. It can be composed of many activities and orchestrated any way you want. Diversify your workouts, otherwise you're likely to get bored. The mind, as well as the body, needs to remain stimulated. It craves more direct involvement. It needs goals and definitive objectives. Your mind, not your body, is what causes you to lose interest in an exercise program. Therefore, before you can initiate change, you must change your thinking patterns.

Another advantage to variety conditioning is that it can reduce injuries by preventing the "overuse syndrome." John Pagliano, a sports medicine podiatrist at Long Beach Memorial Medical Center, says, "Cross training appears to cut down injuries, because various muscle groups are strengthened by the different forms of exercise."

Paddy Calistro[1], in an article for the *Los Angeles Times* on exercising moderation, points out that the ideal cross-training program includes activities that fall into different categories that work different muscles, providing stretching, strengthening, and aerobic portions—sometimes all on the same day and sometimes on alternate days. The idea is to select a few exercises that you actually enjoy and to vary your workouts day to day so that you don't burn out on any one of them.

The following are examples of how a beginning, intermediate, and advanced variety conditioning program might be set up. No two programs are alike. Each depends on a person's goals, interests, and present level of fitness. Here are some examples.

Beginning Variety Conditioning

Frequency: 3 times per week
Duration: 20 to 30 minutes or as tolerated
Intensity: 60 percent to 80 percent Maximal Heart Rate (MHR) or as tolerated (Refer to MHR chart in Chapter 3, page 30 to determine your MHR)
Monday: Exercise program
Tuesday:
Wednesday: Low-impact aerobics, swimming, or tennis
Thursday:
Friday:
Saturday: A brisk walk or cycling
Sunday:

Table I-3

VARIETY CONDITIONING

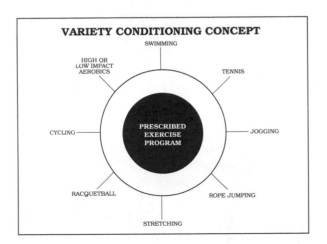

Intermediate Variety Conditioning

Frequency: 4 times per week
Duration: 30 to 45 minutes or as tolerated
Intensity: 65 percent to 80 percent MHR or as tolerated
Monday: Low-impact aerobics or cycling
Tuesday:
Wednesday: Exercise program
Thursday:
Friday: Stretch, rope jump, and jog
Saturday:
Sunday: Tennis or racquetball

Advanced Variety Conditioning

Frequency: 5 to 6 times per week
Duration: Minimum of 45 minutes or as tolerated
Intensity: 70 percent to 85 percent MHR or as tolerated
Monday: Exercise program
Tuesday: Aquatic program or run
Wednesday: Jazzercise, ballet, or aerobics class
Thursday: Exercise program
Friday:
Saturday: Weight-training program or tennis
Sunday: Cycling and rowing machine

Conclusion: Variety conditioning is an option you may want to "exercise." It is not a rigid approach, but rather one of "flexibility," which allows you to make changes or modifications as you see fit. So be creative and go for it! After all, the only thing that success and failure have in common is that they both show that you're trying.

Goals

The Luna Method is based on setting up realistic goals. Knowing what you want and planning how to get it will enable you to reach your goals much sooner and prevent you from wandering around in a maze trying to "find yourself." If your program doesn't have short-term, intermediary, or long-term goals, the probability of success decreases. Write down your goals and date them. This gives you something specific to work for, rather than just "floating" from day to day. Work with visualization and imagery, for what you can conceive, you can achieve. Remember, clarity of vision spells power and success.

Warm-up

The warm-up should consist of a minimum of 10 minutes of light jogging, stretching, and calisthenics. Jog 3 to 5 minutes prior to stretching to facilitate the stretch response. Follow the stretching with a few limbering exercises that slowly imitate the upcoming activity. Never jump into any exercise or activity "cold."

The purpose of the warm-up is to (1) expand the arteries to increase blood flow (arterial vasodilation); (2) increase body temperature; (3) decrease risk of injury; (4) prevent ST-segment depression (abnormal heartbeat[2]), (5) prepare mentally.

Warm-down

The primary purpose of the warm-down is to prevent "blood pooling." During aerobic activity, blood distributes throughout the body, and its return to the heart is assisted by the movement of the muscles. If you remain in the vertical position when you stop exercising, the blood pools in the warm, dilated leg veins. If the person is untrained, the veins lack the ability to contract as effectively as those in a well-trained person. The muscles are no longer pumping the blood back to the heart and ventilation is no longer doing as much to assist venous return (blood vessels that return blood back to the heart). Consequently, the blood accumulates in the legs, with a drastic fall in blood pressure.[3] Perfusion-related symptoms such as dizziness, arrhythmias, or nausea may also result.[4] Therefore, after you finish exercising, walk around for a few minutes to prevent "blood pooling."

"NO PAIN, NO GAIN." FACT OR MYTH?

The Luna Method is not associated with the "no pain, no gain" concept. Over the past twenty years, I have been particularly disturbed by the proliferation of this phrase. Some fitness "experts" extol the necessity of associated pain with exercise if "gains" are to be made. This phrase is constantly pounded into the heads of budding and prospective exercise enthusiasts in books, magazines, television, and films. My answer to "no pain, no gain" is that it is medically unsound advice.

The concept was never intended for the average person who decides to start an exercise program, structured or otherwise. If you know you're going to be in pain every time you exercise, are you going to want to do it? Will you stretch if you know in doing so you're going to be in pain? Or will you run if you feel pain? I know for a few, pain is tolerated and accepted as part of the exercise program. What has happened, unfortunately, is that many people have been brainwashed into believing that pain must be felt if any benefits are to be derived from exercise. Train instead at a pace or level that is well tolerated. Otherwise, the likelihood of continuing with the program on a long-term basis would appear to be unlikely.

Let's talk about pain for a moment. Pain has two very distinct functions, one negative and one positive. The negative side of pain is that it hurts. I'm sure a few of you may be thinking, how can pain have a positive function if it hurts? Well, in the process of hurting, it also lets your body know that something is not right. Pain acts as a warning system, a defense mechanism. Your body talks to you through pain and other senses. Unfortunately, many people don't acknowledge pain. The body protects itself and allows it to heal through an awareness of pain. It's when we don't listen to pain that we get into trouble. It's when your knees are killing you and you go out and run those two or three miles anyway because you feel you just have to do it that you'll end up regretting it later. Keep this in mind: it's not how hard you train; it's how intelligently you train that matters.

The only people who may apply the no pain, no gain concept are world-class and professional athletes. When I work with elite athletes, there is going to be pain, but it's for another reason. Because most of these athletes are at a fitness level where rigorous and intensive training can be tolerated, there's a difference in the purpose and objective for the pain.

Use the following guidelines (not pain) to determine your progress:

1. Increase in endurance
2. Increase in strength
3. Increase in flexibility
4. Decrease in body fat
5. Decrease in resting heart rate
6. Decrease in weight, where needed
7. Improvement in appearance and health

Always train within your target heart rates and remember that everything you do should always be done as tolerated.

A WORD ABOUT BURNOUT

The Luna Method is not involved and does not have anything to do with overtraining, which could subsequently lead to "burnout." Burnout is defined as physical, mental, or emotional exhaustion as related to a certain stimulus, in this case, exercise. Sometimes there's a tendency to

get so caught up with training caused by a perfectionist attitude, abnormal need in improving performance, or breaking a record, personal or otherwise, that you neglect to listen to your body when it tells you it needs a break. To spot and avoid this condition, be aware of the following physical, mental, and emotional signs:

Physical Signs

1. Listlessness
2. Low energy
3. Chronic fatigue
4. Weakness
5. Muscle soreness
6. Decreased level of resistance
7. Difficulty sleeping

Mental Signs

1. Loss of motivation
2. Negative attitude
3. Poor self-image
4. Indifference
5. Worthlessness
6. Blaming others
7. Pessimism
8. Resistance toward training
9. Conflicting personality
10. Psychosomatic illnesses

Emotional Signs

1. Depression
2. Hopelessness
3. Irritability
4. Nervousness
5. Dissatisfaction
6. Loneliness
7. Discouragement
8. Disenchantment
9. Lack of coping mechanisms

If you find yourself "burning out," there are several ways of controlling the condition: (a) Recognize that you have "burnout." (b) Decrease frequency, intensity, and duration of activity. (c) Re-establish priorities, and learn when to say "no." If you overload, you're going to be right back where you started. (d) Accept that which you can and cannot change. (e) Learn from the situation. (f) Compartmentalize: make a separation between one task and another. For example, when you get home from work, imagine as you undress you're shedding the day's problems. (g) Find a support group or a close friend who will listen. (h) Write down how you feel in a journal.

If you continue to have a problem with "burnout," seek professional counseling. The one positive thing that could be said about "burnout" is that it could serve as a catalyst for change.

CHAPTER 1 NOTES

[1] Calistro, Paddy, "Exercising Moderation," *Los Angeles Times,* January 18, 1987, p. 28.

[2] R.J. Barnard, R. McAlpin, A.A. Kattus, *et al,* "Ischemic Responses to Sudden Strenuous Exercise in Healthy Men," *Circulation,* Vol. 48, November 1973, pp. 936-942.

[3] Shephard, Roy J., "Exercise and the Cardiovascular System," *The Physician and Sportsmedicine,* Vol. 7, No. 9, September 1979, p. 57.

[4] Zohman, L.R., *Beyond Diet: Exercise Your Way to Fitness and Heart Health* (Englewood Cliffs, New Jersey: CPC International, Inc., 1974).

Chapter 2

STRETCHING

Inflexible thinking is incapable of adaptability and pliability. The truth lies beyond inflexible thoughts.

—David Luna

A few years back, I was working with Eddie Bell of the New York Jets. He had just been traded to the Green Bay Packers and came to see me that summer for a conditioning program. I put him on a weight-training program to build up his lean body mass (muscle) and increase his strength. Since he was a wide receiver, I also had him on a running, rope-jumping, and stretching program. He followed it regularly, with the exception of the stretching. When it came time for him to leave for camp, I wished him well, still unaware that he had not done any stretching. He had gotten himself into excellent condition, but he was tight as a knot. For a wide receiver to be tight is dangerous. This position requires speed, agility, strength, endurance, explosiveness, and flexibility. As you might have predicted, when he got to camp to begin his training, he pulled one muscle after another. Three weeks later, he was back in Los Angeles and out of a job.

Stretching is an integral part of all the fitness and training programs we teach at Fitness Professionals of America. Its purpose is threefold: (1) reduce the risk of injury; (2) increase flexibility; and (3) increased range of motion. Stretching should be practiced before and after all workouts.

In all the years I've been training and competing, I've never started a workout without doing a minimum of five minutes of stretching. If I don't personally stretch out clients, I have them stretch independently before and after all workouts.

Unfortunately, many people don't believe in stretching. Very often I observe runners come out on the track and start running without doing any stretching. I see tennis and racquetball players jump onto the court without stretching. I notice many body builders and weight lifters walk into a gym and "warm up" by bench pressing a couple hundred pounds. From my perspective, that's too risky and short-sighted. When you compare the risks versus the benefits, there's no comparison. The benefits of stretching by far outweigh the risks of not stretching. Always think long-term. If you want to have a lengthy and active athletic career, I strongly suggest that you stretch on a daily basis.

Flexibility is specific to each joint, and therefore specific stretching exercises are needed to improve inflexible areas. Limited flexibility is usually the result of muscles and tendons that are too tight, which in some cases may restrict range of motion.

19

Why are some people less flexible than others? The following reasons are generally accepted by health professionals as the probable causes of poor or limited flexibility:

1. Genetics—some people are born with less flexibility than others; not that the muscles are less flexible, but as a result of tighter joints and shorter muscles and tendons, flexibility is harder to obtain.
2. Lack of stretching—if you don't stretch on a regular basis, it's difficult to maintain muscular and connective-tissue flexibilty and pliability.
3. Improper stretching—there are many ways of stretching incorrectly, but two common mistakes frequently made are bouncing and stretching to the point of pain.
4. Dysfunction syndrome—this condition refers to adaptive shortening of muscle or connective tissues for a variety of reasons; a common one relates to injuries, which produce adhesions (scars) that may form on areas such as the back, shoulders, elbows, and knees.
5. Combination of any or all of these.

Stretching exercises should be performed statically and not ballistically. Static stretching involves a slow, controlled stretching movement followed by holding the functional stretch for approximately thirty seconds. Static stretching reduces the risk of injury and promotes relaxation of the muscles involved in the stretch. Ballistic stretching involves forced, bouncing movements in which the "functional stretch" is not held. Ballistic stretching should be avoided as it may cause microtears to the muscle or muscles being stretched.

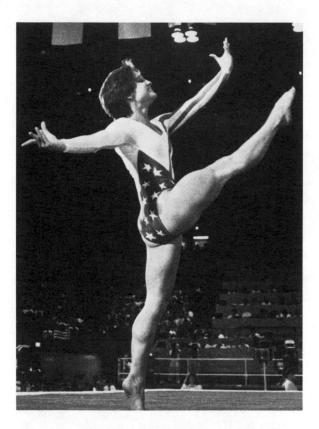

Figure 2-1. Mary Lou Retton, Olympic Gymnast and Gold Medalist; 1984 Olympics. *(Reprinted with permission of the* Los Angeles Times *copyright 1984.)*

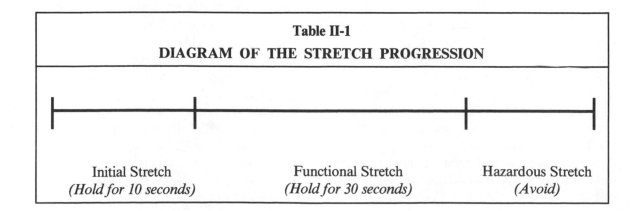

Table II-1

DIAGRAM OF THE STRETCH PROGRESSION

Initial Stretch	Functional Stretch	Hazardous Stretch
(Hold for 10 seconds)	*(Hold for 30 seconds)*	*(Avoid)*

Stretching is easy to learn and enjoyable if you don't force the stretching. The most important aspect of stretching is to learn to stretch within your limits. There should be no pain associated with stretching. Forcing a stretch beyond your limit is self-defeating and delays your progress. When you force a stretch, it not only causes pain and possible injury, but it also inhibits the stretch response of the muscle fibers. When you overstretch a muscle, it automatically contracts (the opposite of what you're trying to achieve). It does this as a defense mechanism to protect itself from being torn or injured.

When you begin a stretch, slowly stretch to the point of a gentle pull and hold it for

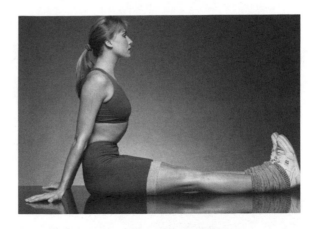

Figure 2-3. Keep feet dorsiflexed (toes pointed towards you) unless indicated otherwise.

approximately ten seconds. The first part of the stretch is called the "initial stretch" (see Table II-1). As the tension from the initial stretch subsides, slowly and gently stretch into the "functional stretch" and hold for approximately thirty seconds. The functional stretch increases flexibility. You should feel a slight pull, but not pain. After thirty seconds, release the functional stretch gently. Avoid stretching into the "hazardous" stretching position. This stretch is generally characterized by pain or a quivering in the lower or upper extremity as a result of being overstretched.

When stretching, your breathing should be natural and rhythmical. Do not hold your breath. Also, set a goal for each stretch, and remember, always stretch within your limits. If you're very tight in a specific area, place more time and emphasis on that region.

The following recommendations will help you to improve your stretching and to progress at a much faster rate:

1. Keep in mind that stretching is a way to relax and become more in tune with your body.
2. Maintain slow and rhythmic breathing to help in relaxation and to stretch more effectively.
3. Keep your feet dorsiflexed (toes pointed toward you), unless otherwise indicated.
4. Hold each stretch for approximately thirty

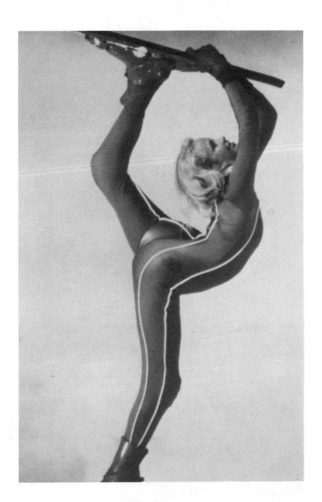

Figure 2-2. Suzy Chaffee, the "First Lady of Skiing," Olympic Alpine ski star, and three-time World Freestyle Ski Champion. Do not attempt this stretch. *(Photo by Robert Troxello.)*

seconds or count to ten very slowly.

5. Move gently and gracefully from one stretch to the next. Avoid abrupt movements.

6. Set goals for each stretch and visualize yourself reaching those goals.

7. Be patient with yourself. You don't become flexible overnight. Continuous practice will allow you to come closer and closer to your goals.

8. Stretch before and after all workouts.

9. Try not to stretch to the point of pain. A gentle pull is okay, but there should be *no* pain associated with stretching.

10. Don't hold your breath during any stretch. Doing so may produce an immediate rise in blood pressure and cause dizziness, particularly with weight-bearing exercises.

11. Don't rush. Stretching is a slow, relaxing process, which should not be associated with pressure, tension, or anxiety.

12. Don't bounce. Bouncing produces small muscle tears and causes the muscles to contract, which is the opposite of what you're trying to do.

13. Try not to expect too much too soon. Be aware of the difference between the gentle pull of a comfortable stretch and the pain that may result when you have stretched too far.

14. Don't make comparisons with others. Competition never works here.

15. Try not to place a great deal of emphasis on flexibility in the beginning, rather, on how the stretch *feels*. Any attempt to overcompensate for the lack of flexibility will work against you. Let your body lead you slowly and naturally into its full potential of flexibility.

FLEXIBILITY EXERCISES

The following stretches are to increase flexibility and range of motion in areas that are commonly tight:

Knee to Chest Stretch

Lie on your back. Grasp your right knee and gently pull towards your chest. Hold the stretch for about 30 seconds or a slow count of 10. Return slowly to the starting position and switch to the opposite side. In this and all of the following stretches, please do not take any stretch to the point of pain. (See Figure 2-4.)

Double Knee to Chest

Lie on your back. Grasp both knees and gently pull toward your chest. Hold for

Figure 2-4. Knee to Chest.

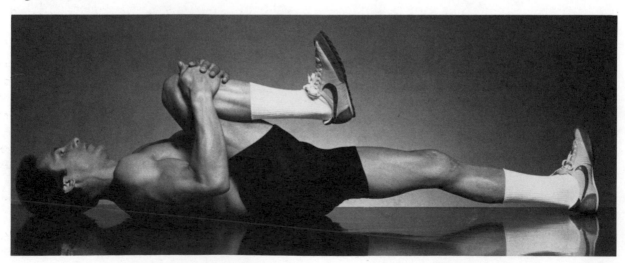

approximately 30 seconds or a slow count of 10. As always, keep your feet dorsiflexed. (See Figure 2-5.)

Seated Forward Stretch

Sit with your feet together, legs extended. Slowly and gently bend forward at the waist. Hold on to your knees, calves, ankles, or feet. A slight bend of the knees is all right. If you have difficulty in stretching forward, use a rolled-up towel to assist you. Holding on to both ends, place the middle part of the towel under your feet. (See Figure 2-6.)

"V" Stretch

Open legs as wide as possible into a "V" position. Keep your feet dorsiflexed. Gently reach over and stretch to your right. As you stretch to your right, keep your left hip grounded. It will have a tendency to lift from the floor. Hold for approximately 30 seconds and repeat on the opposite side. (See Figure 2-7.)

Diamond Stretch

Sit with your legs apart and feet dorsiflexed. Gently hold on to your knees, calves, ankles, or feet as you slowly stretch forward. (See Figure 2-8.)

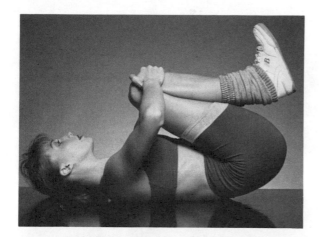

Figure 2-5. Double Knee to Chest.

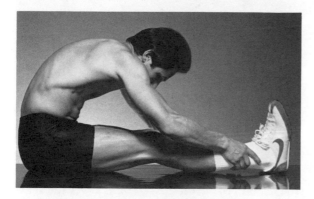

Figure 2-6. Seated Forward Stretch.

Figure 2-7. "V" Stretch.

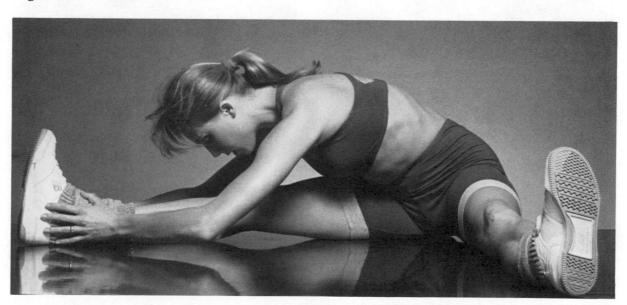

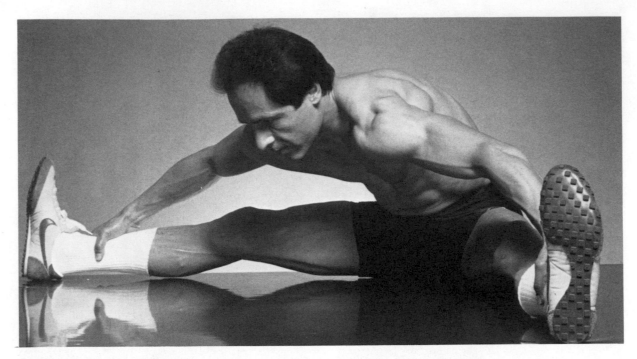

Figure 2-8. Diamond Stretch.

Figure 2-9. Half Hurdler.

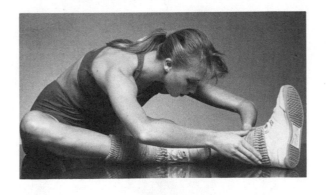

Half Hurdler

From a seated position, extend the left leg and partially bend your right leg about halfway. Gently stretch in the direction of the extended leg. Make sure to keep the right hip grounded and keep the bent knee as close to the floor as possible. Maintain rhythmic breathing and hold for 30 seconds. Repeat on the opposite side. (See Figure 2-9.)

Beginning Butterfly

Sit with knees turned out, feet together, and back straight. Holding feet together with both hands, pull the chest upward and lower the knees as close to the floor as possible. (See Figure 2-10.)

Advanced Butterfly

Sit with knees turned out and feet together. Holding feet with both hands, lower knees to the ground, and bring the forehead as close to the feet as possible. (See Figure 2-11.)

Knee-over

Lie on your back and lift right knee to chest. Place left hand on the outside of the right knee and pull it gently across your body. Bring the bent knee as close to the floor as possible. If you want to stretch the middle and lower back, bring knee above the waistline. If you want more of a lower back stretch, bring knee below the waistline. Turn your head to the right and keep both shoulders grounded. Repeat on the opposite side. (See Figure 2-12.)

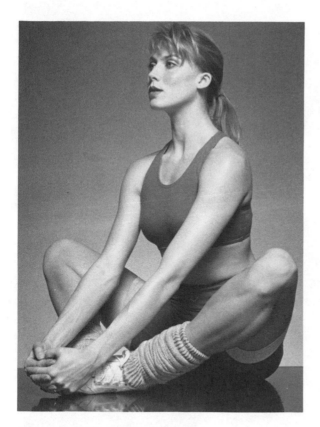

Figure 2-10. Beginning Butterfly.

Figure 2-11. Advanced Butterfly.

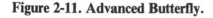

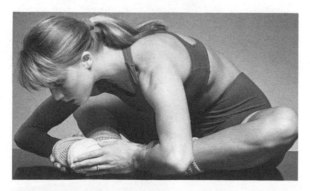

Figure 2-12. Knee-over.

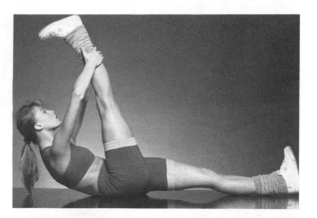

Figure 2-13. Right Angle Stretch.

Figure 2-14. Foot to Forehead.

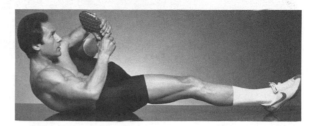

Right Angle Stretch

Lie on your back, hands at your sides and feet together. Raise right leg up, either straight or slightly bent. Grasp with both hands the back of the knee, calf, ankle, or foot, and gently pull knee towards forehead. Hold for 30 seconds. Repeat on opposite side. (See Figure 2-13.)

Foot to Forehead

Lie on your back. Grasp left foot with both hands and gently bring foot as close as possible to forehead. Repeat on opposite side. (See Figure 2-14.)

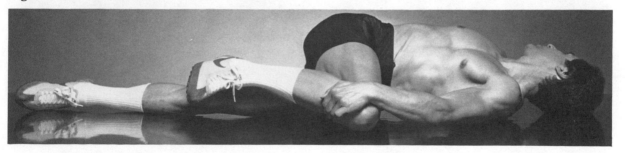

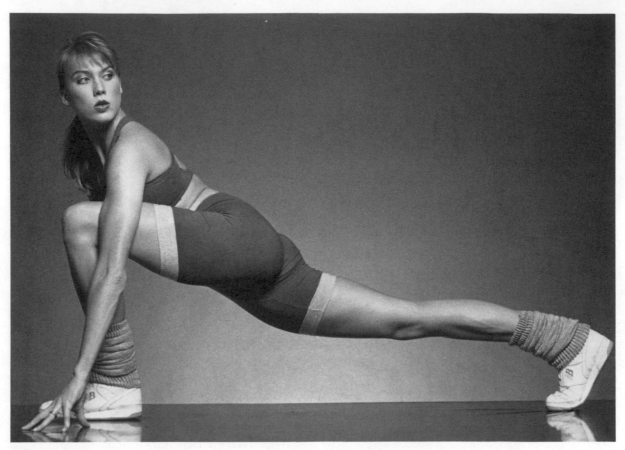

Figure 2-15. Forward Lunge.

Forward Lunge

Lunge forward with left leg, keeping right leg straight. Left foot should be directly below left knee. Place hands on floor for balance and look backwards over left shoulder. Repeat on the opposite side. (See Figure 2-15.)

Knee-bow Stretch

Starting position is on your hands and knees. Shift your weight back while simultaneously stretching your arms and shoulders forward. Hold for 30 seconds. This should be avoided if you have sensitive knees. (See Figure 2-16.)

Figure 2-16. Kneel-Bow Stretch.

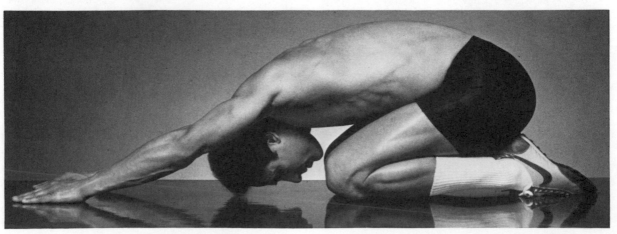

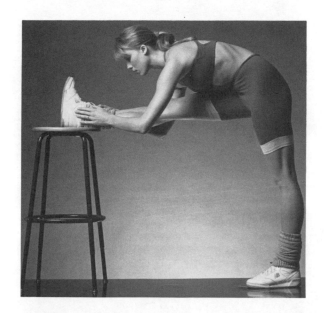

Ballet Bar Stretch

Place your right foot on a stable support so that your leg can extend straight out in front of you. Keep your right foot dorsiflexed. Gently bend forward as you either hold on to your knee, calf, ankle, or foot. Concentrate on bringing the forehead towards your knee. Do not attempt to prop your foot on a surface that is too high. (See Figure 2-17.)

Figure 2-17. Ballet Bar Stretch.

Calf Stretch

Stand facing a wall approximately 3 to 4 feet away. Lean forward and place both hands on the wall. Place left foot behind your right knee. As you lean foward, keep the right heel grounded. If you are unable to do so, move closer to the wall. If you don't feel any stretch in the calf, move your right foot back a little more. Also, keep your body straight throughout the stretch. Repeat on the opposite side. (See Figure 2-18.)

Achilles Tendon Stretch

Follow the identical instructions that you would for the Calf Stretch, with one exception: Bend the right leg slightly. (See Figure 2-19.)

Posterior Cuff Stretch

Place left hand over your right elbow and bring the right arm across your chest. Keep the right arm straight and turn your head to the right. Hold for 30 seconds. Repeat on the other side. (See Figure 2-20.)

Figure 2-18. Calf Stretch.

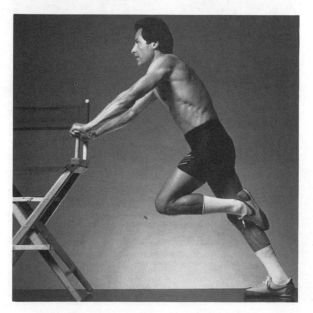

Figure 2-19. Achilles Tendon Stretch.

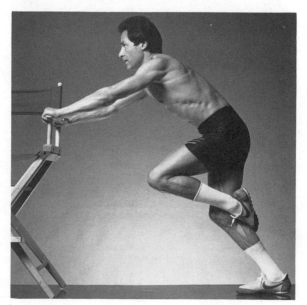

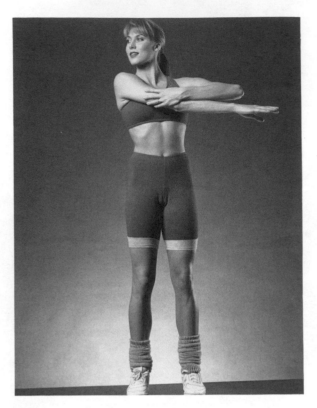

Figure 2-20. Posterior Cuff Stretch.

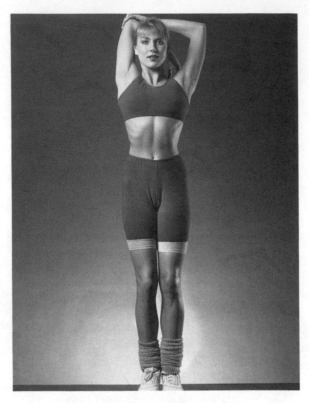

Figure 2-21. Inferior Cuff Stretch.

Inferior Cuff Stretch

Elevate bent right arm above your head. Hold on to the right elbow with the left hand for approximately 30 seconds. Repeat on the opposite side. Variation: this stretch could also be done by holding both elbows simultaneously. (See Figure 2-21.)

Highbar Stretch

If a highbar is available, hang for approximately 20 to 30 seconds. This is an excellent stretch for shoulders, lats, and back. (See Figure 2-22.)

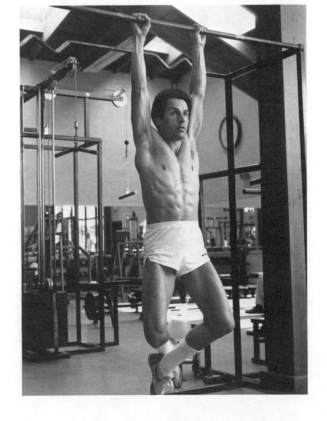

Figure 2-22. Highbar Stretch.

Chapter 3

AEROBIC EXERCISE AND HEART RATE

Much of the human deterioration that we attribute to aging is simply a manifestation of the deconditioning effect caused by inactivity.

—Laurence Morehouse

Activities that increase cardiovascular fitness are called aerobics. Aerobic exercises include— but are not limited to— walking, running, rope-jumping, cycling, swimming, rowing, and cross-country skiing. By regularly participating in one or more of these aerobic activities, you may do any or all of these things:

1. Decrease body fat
2. Lose weight
3. Increase endurance
4. Strengthen your heart
5. Lower cholesterol and triglycerides (fats in the blood)
6. Improve muscle tone
7. Reduce stress
8. Lower blood pressure[1]
9. Improve diabetic conditions through weight-reduction and improved glucose use[2]
10. Retard the progression of osteoporosis— fragile and brittle bones[3]
11. Improve coordination, mechanical efficiency, and strength[4]
12. Improve self-esteem
13. Improve sleep patterns and bowel functions[5]

To determine appropriate aerobic activity, or more specifically the level of intensity, use "target heart rates." Target heart rates enable you to determine how much exercise is too much as well as not enough. As a general rule, aerobic capacity will improve if exercise is of sufficient intensity to increase heart rate to about 70 percent of maximum.[6] It should also be pointed out that exercise does not need to be strenuous in order to obtain positive results. Remember the old axiom of "no pain, no gain" is medically unsound advice.

There are several ways to determine appropriate target heart rates. The first method to determine your target heart rate for maximum benefit and safety is to start with the number 220 (for males) and 226 (for females), subtract your age, then multiply by .70. For example, a forty-year-old man in average condition would use the following equation:

$$220 - 40 \times .70 = 126 \text{ BPM (beats per minute)}$$

The second method to determine recommended exercise heart rates is through the use of the Average Maximal Heart Rates chart shown on Table III-1. First, locate your age, using the

				Table III-1				
			AVERAGE MAXIMAL HEART RATES*					
Age	*MAX H.R.*	*90% MHR*	*85% MHR*	*80% MHR*	*75% MHR*	*70% MHR*	*65% MHR*	*60% MHR*
25	190	171	162	152	143	133	124	114
30	186	167	158	149	140	130	121	112
35	182	164	155	146	137	127	118	109
40	181	163	154	145	136	127	118	109
45	179	161	152	143	134	125	116	107
50	175	158	149	140	131	123	114	105
55	171	154	145	137	128	120	111	103
60	168	151	143	134	126	118	109	101
65	164	148	139	131	123	115	107	98

From "The National Workshop on Exercise in the Prevention, in the Evolution, and in the Treatment of Heart Disease," J.S. Carolina Medical Association, *Vol. 65, Supplement 1, Dec. 1969.*

column on the far left. The numbers to the right of the age column are the average maximal heart rates. If you exercise regularly and are in good condition, maintain an exercise heart rate between 70 percent and 85 percent for a minimum of twenty minutes, if possible. If you are not in good cardiovascular condition, maintain an exercise heart rate between 60 percent and 75 percent. Two good rules of thumb to remember are: (1) All exercise should be done as tolerated. (2) You should be able to carry on a conversation while exercising. If you're unable to do so, you are exercising too strenuously. For example, if you're thirty-five years of age and are exercising on a regular basis, your recommended exercise heart rate is between 127 and 155 BPM. If you are under 127 BPM while exercising, you can pick up the tempo. Conversely, if you are over 155 BPM while exercising, slow down.

These figures are nothing more than safe training parameters for a person thirty-five years of age. The figures will vary according to age. Therefore, refer to Table III-1 to determine your specific exercise heart rates.

To produce cardiovascular benefit and fitness, the stimulus period should include 20 to 60 minutes of continuous exercise without stopping, except to monitor the pulse.[7] To achieve metabolic benefits of exercise, such as improved carbohydrate tolerance and blood lipid profile (fat, cholesterol, etc.), the exercise duration should be 20 minutes or longer.[8] Keep two things in mind with regards to cardiovascular exercise: (1) The average person is not going to be able to do 20 minutes of continuous activity initially; 5 to 10 minutes might be more practical and realistic. (2) Start out gradually and moderately with whatever you can do comfortably; if you start getting tired, stop and rest; you'll be able to do a little more next time.

You will find that activity sustained during exercise conditions will eventually produce a decrease in heart rate under rest conditions. Many marathon runners, for example, have resting heart rates in the 50s or 60s. I'm not a marathon runner, but through cardiovascular conditioning, I've been able to lower my resting pulse rate to 48 beats per minutes. You can do the same, and by doing so, decrease the workload on your heart.

Table III-2 will give you an idea of normal resting pulse rates, expressed in beats per minute.

Keep in mind that these are average rates under rest conditions.

Tachycardia (abnormally rapid heart rate under rest conditions) and bradycardia (slow heartbeat under rest conditions) are terms used to refer to heart rates at either end of the continuum. Tachycardia is a heart rate over 100 BPM at rest and is undesirable. Bradycardia is a heart rate of less that 60 BPM at rest and is considered desirable. A slow heart rate is generally representative of physical fitness, that is, if it is achieved by exercise.

Table III-2	
NORMAL RESTING PULSE RATES	
Men	72-76 BPM
Women	75-80 BPM
Boys	80-84 BPM
Girls	82-89 BPM

Pulse rate changes throughout the day. Events, stress, tension, anxiety, and caffeine or other stimulants all have an effect on heart rate. In general, though, heart rate is lowest during sleep and increases about 5 to 10 beats during the day.

Pulse rate is one of the best measures of physical fitness. A well-conditioned individual has a slow increase in heart rate upon exercising and a rapid recovery rate upon termination, whereas an individual in poor condition has a rapid increase in heart rate upon exercising, and a slow, gradual recovery rate upon termination.

USING PULSE RATE TO MONITOR YOUR FITNESS

There are several areas where the pulsation of the heart can be felt. The radial artery is the most common. If light pressure is applied with both the index and middle fingers, at the position indicated, usually pulsation can be felt. If you have difficulty finding the radial artery, try the

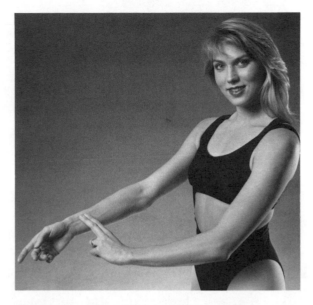

Figure 3-1. Using Pulse Rate to Monitor Your Fitness.

Figure 3-2.

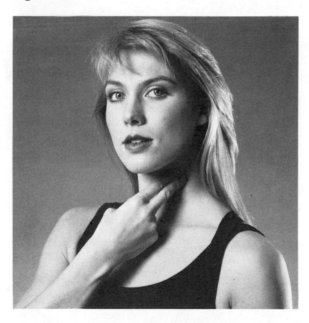

carotid artery in the neck. The pulsation there is usually strong and easy to find. Apply light pressure below the lower jaw, but do not compress both sides simultaneously. Once you locate your pulse, count the number of beats for 10 seconds and multiply by 6. This will give you the heart rate for 1 minute. (See Figures 3-1 and 3-2.)

Pharmacologic Medications that Affect Heart Rate in Cardiac Patients[9]

The following medications may either increase or decrease resting heart rate:

1. Antianginal medications such as Nitroglycerin (increase heart rate)
2. Beta blockers such as Inderal, Lopressor, or Tenormin (decrease heart rate)
3. Calcium channel blockers such as Procardia (increase heart rate), Cardizem (decrease heart rate), or Calan (decrease heart rate)
4. High blood pressure medications such as Minipress (increase heart rate), Catapres (decrease heart rate), or Apresoline (increase heart rate)
5. Antiarrhythmics such as Lanoxin (decrease heart rate)

CHAPTER 3 NOTES

[1] Wheat, Mary E., "Exercise in the Elderly," *The Western Journal of Medicine,* October 1987, Vol. 147, No. 4, p. 477.

[2] *Ibid.*

[3] *Ibid.*

[4] *Ibid.*

[5] *Ibid.*

[6] McArdle, William D.; Katch, Frank; and Katch, Victor, *Exercise Physiology, Energy, Nutrition, and Human Performance* (Philadelphia: Lea & Febiger, 1981), p. 274.

[7] S. Gibson, S. Gerberich, A. Leon, "Writing the Exercise Prescription: An Individualized Approach," *The Physician and Sportsmedicine,* Vol. 11, No. 7, July 1983.

[8] *Guidelines for Exercise Testing and Prescription,* American College of Sports Medicine (Philadelphia: Lea & Febiger, 1986), pp. 148-152.

[9]. *Ibid.*

Chapter 4

BEGINNING, INTERMEDIATE, AND ADVANCED WORKOUTS

Happy are those who dream dreams and are ready to pay the price to make them come true.

—L.J. Cardinal Suenes

Having been involved in the health profession most of my life, there are certain questions that I and many of my colleagues are asked on a frequent basis. One of these involves recommending exercises for specific body parts. Everyone has different problem areas—some major and some minor. But regardless of the degree of necessity or neglect, all 650 muscles in your body need to be worked.

It is as a result of this need that I have developed a series of beginning, intermediate, and advanced exercises to assist you in zeroing in on major problem areas. In addition, the program will enable you to keep your weight down, while preventing demoralizing sights such as "fanny fallout," "midsection mismanagement," "angel wings," and "thunder thighs."

Exercise at whatever level you feel is best suited for you. The first week, start with the beginning exercises only. After the first week, progress gradually as tolerated. Don't be surprised if you find yourself working at different levels. For example, you may find the beginning shoulder exercise difficult, while finding the advanced abdominal exercise "just right." This is quite normal. Everyone has different strengths and weaknesses, which will vary as a result of genetics, lifestyles, fitness history, or other factors. Build a solid foundation before moving up to the intermediate and advanced exercise levels.

If you're at a beginning or intermediate level, rest in between exercises and monitor your heart rate. If you're at an advanced level, you have one of two options: (1) limit your rest periods to approximately 30 seconds or (2) if well tolerated, you can go from one exercise to another without rest, unless intermittent pulse checks indicate your exercise pulse rate is too high; if that's the case, then either slow down or stop.

Your program will cover all the major muscle groups. It will also give you the opportunity to spend more time working on those problem areas that you feel require more time and attention. Two words of caution: (a) Avoid any exercise that causes pain or discomfort to areas such as the back, knees, shoulders, and elbows. (b) Do not become obsessed with perfecting one body part at the expense of another; work all areas; neglect none; and emphasize your weaknesses. The key is *balance*.

The recommendations for the prescribed exercise program are as shown in Table IV-1.

Table IV-1
A BALANCED EXERCISE PROGRAM
FREQUENCY: 3 times per week initially; you may increase gradually as your level of fitness improves.
REPETITIONS: 12-15 times, or as tolerated
DURATION: 20-30 minutes, or as tolerated
INTENSITY: In general, keep your pulse between 120 and 150 BPM; see Table III-1 for specific figures.

The following is an example of how the prescribed exercise program may be set up in conjunction with the variety conditioning concept for someone at an intermediate level:

Monday: Low-impact aerobics
Tuesday:
Wednesday: Prescribed exercise program
Thursday:
Friday: Tennis or racquetball
Saturday: Stretch
Sunday: Prescribed exercise program

How Long Before I See Results?

As a rule, tune-ups take about 7 to 10 days; rear end alignments normally take about 3 to 6 months; major overhauls average about 1 to 2 years.

Seriously, I cannot answer that question fully, nor could anyone else. There are just too many variables involved. Instead, concentrate on seeing some type of improvement over a period of time. Subtle changes will occur initially. Pronounced

changes will take place as you get more into the program on a regular basis. For example, if you see your weight dropping or you notice an increase in strength and endurance, or an improvement in muscle tonicity, then you know you're moving in the right direction. When you stand in front of a mirror in your birthday suit, doing a 360 degree turn, you'll see what areas need work. When your clothes start getting looser on you, assuming you want to lose weight, you'll know you're moving in the right direction. Don't get hung up on length of time, but rather on day-to-day, week-to-week, month-to-month improvement or attainment of your goals.

How Often Should I Revise My Prescribed Exercise Program?

Ideally, exercise programs should be revised approximately every ninety days. There are several reasons for this. First of all, any program that is done for an extended period of time is extremely limiting. There are endless ways to work the body, but being the creatures of habit that we are, we have a tendency to embrace a particular set of exercises that we feel comfortable with. Secondly, doing the same exercises the same number of times over and over is boring. Program revisions keep the interest level up; therefore, feel free to add new exercises, set goals, increase the degree of difficulty, decrease rest periods, and make modifications whenever you see fit. Avoid complacency, shun ruts, and keep improving. It can always be better!

Spot Reducing

Many people are under the impression that if you concentrate on exercising an obese part of the body, you'll reduce it. Unfortunately, it doesn't work this way. There is no such thing as "spot reducing." For example, doing lots of sit-ups is not going to reduce a protruding mid-section. If you attempt to counteract an over-weight problem by concentrating solely on one anatomical area without making any dietary changes or working the entire body, your chances of being successful will probably not be very good. Basically all that you're doing is solidifying muscle mass underneath a layer of fat.

What's so frustrating to most people is that the areas they want to lose the most are generally the last to go. So don't waste your time doing hundreds of sit-ups every day to eradicate a flabby midsection, unless you are planning to enter a sit-up contest. Yes, you'll burn calories by doing lots of sit ups, but you're also going to get very bored and very sore. Instead, concentrate on integrating activities that utilize large muscle groups (legs, chest, and back) and are of sustained duration, such as walking, cycling, and swimming, in conjunction with your prescribed abdominal exercises, to burn as many calories as possible. Simultaneously, practice Systematic Undereating and Behavioral Modification as outlined in Chapter 7.

POTENTIALLY HAZARDOUS EXERCISES

The following exercises have been determined to be potentially hazardous by Fitness Professionals of America and should be avoided:

1. Plow
2. Standing toe touches
3. Hurdler stretch
4. Lay back hurdler stretch
5. Heel sit/shin stretch
6. Ballistic or forced stretching
7. Fast neck circles
8. Bentover twists with rounded back
9. Whipping or swinging movements
10. Straight leg sit-ups
11. Straight leg double leg raises
12. Deep knee bends (90° knee bends are okay)
13. Running with ankle weights
14. Sustained isometric exercises
15. Jack-knifes
16. "Good morning" exercise (90° forward bends with legs straight and a barbell on shoulders)
17. Rear leg lifts above parallel
18. Deadlifts with legs straight.
19. Any exercise that involves lifting with the legs straight and the back rounded. Always keep the knees bent and the back flat when lifting or performing exercises

Before you start your prescribed exercise program, there's a checklist I would like you to go over:

1. Get a medical okay from your family physician.
2. Prep yourself mentally for your workout. Plan out what you want to do and how you want to go about it.
3. Dress the part. Get into exercise clothes that are comfortable.
4. Empty your bladder.
5. If you feel thirsty while exercising, then have a drink. The old myth about not drinking water during exercise was discarded years ago.
6. Wait about one and a half to two hours after you've eaten before you start your workout.
7. Don't socialize until after you've completed your exercise program. It interferes with your concentration.
8. If working out at home, put on the answering machine. If you have a family, put up the "Do not Disturb" sign. Interruptions are too distracting.
9. Exercise on a carpeted area or use a towel or an exercise pad for your floor work.
10. When you're exercising, always exhale on the effort. Never hold your breath.
11. Exercise to music.
12. Listen to your body and take intermittent pulse-rate checks.

Now, you're ready to start!
Your prescribed exercise program will focus on the following muscle regions:

1. Shoulders (deltoids)
2. Back of the arms (triceps)
3. Front of the arms (biceps)

4. Forearms
5. Chest or bustline
6. Upper back
7. Lower back
8. Upper abdominals
9. Lower abdominals
10. Sides of the waist (external obliques)
11. Hips
12. Outer thighs (abductors)
13. Inner thighs (adductors)
14. Front thighs (quadriceps)
15. Back thighs (hamstrings)
16. Calves (gastrocnemius)
17. Shin muscles (anterior tibial muscles)

SHOULDER EXERCISES

Beginning—Reverse Windmills

Extend both arms out, hands pointing upward. Bend both legs slightly and keep your rear end tucked in. Make small circles with both arms in a backward direction. Light wrist weights are optional. *Repetitions:* 20 times or as tolerated. (See Figure 4-1.)

Intermediate—Alternate Dumbbell Presses

Take a couple of light dumbbells. Starting

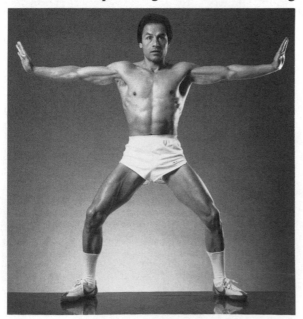

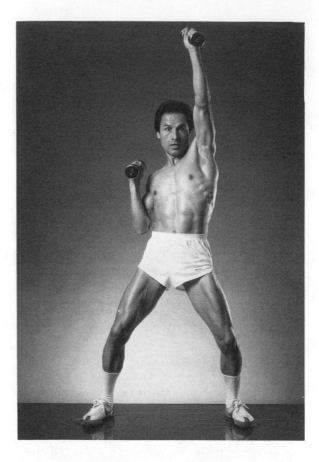

Figure 4-2. Alternate Dumbbell Presses.

position is with the dumbbells at shoulder level. Extend the left arm overhead, then the right. Hold on tightly to both dumbbells. Keep both legs slightly bent. Exhale on the way up; inhale on the way down. *Repetitions:* 10-15 times or as tolerated. (See Figure 4-2.)

Advanced—Shoulder Raise to Side

Using either a pulley or dumbbell, lift the arm laterally until it is parallel to the ground or at shoulder level. Slowly lower the weight, using negative resistance. Avoid inertia and the recovery phase. If done with dumbbells or on a machine, work both arms simultaneously. Exhale on the way up, inhale on the way down. *Repetitions:* 10-15 or as tolerated. (See Figure 4-3.)

Figure 4-1. Reverse Windmills.

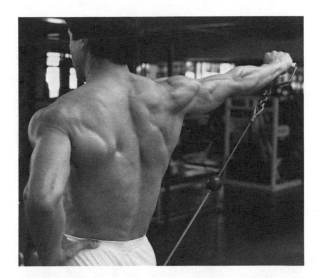

Figure 4-3. Shoulder Raise to Side.

TRICEP EXERCISES

Beginning—Seated Tricep Extensions

Take a light dumbbell and grasp it tightly with both hands. Lift it overhead. Bend your arms behind the head and extend arms fully back to starting position. Keep both elbows as close together as possible to avoid flaring. Inhale on the way down; exhale on the way up. *Repetitions:* 10-15 times or as tolerated. (See Figures 4-4 and 4-5.)

Intermediate— Bentover Tricep Extensions ("Kickbacks")

Take a couple of light dumbbells. Bend your knees and keep your back flat. Extend the arms back until the arms are straight or parallel to the

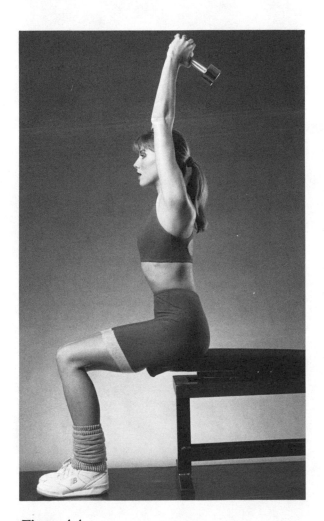

Figure 4-4.

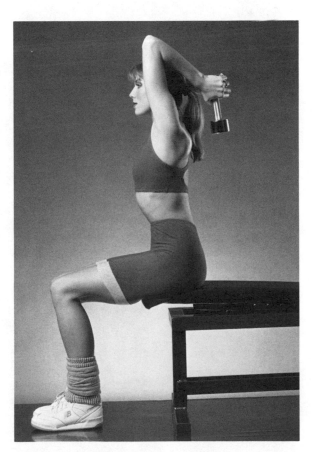

Figure 4-5. Seated Tricep Extensions.

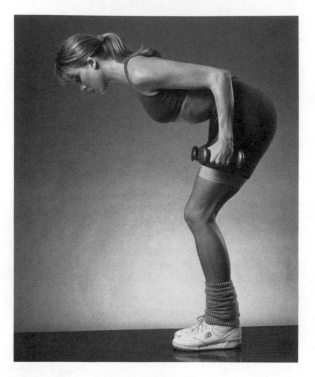

Figure 4-6.

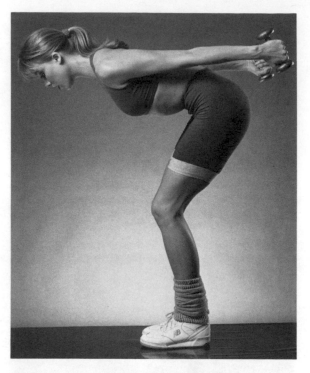

Figure 4-7. Bentover Tricep Extensions.

ground. Limit range of motion to 90 degress or less. Avoid swinging the arms like a pendulum. Exhale as the arms go back; inhale as they come forward. *Repetitions:* 10-15 times or as tolerated. (See Figures 4-6 and 4-7.)

Advanced—Women's Push-ups

Begin on your hands and knees. Place your hands on the floor equidistant to shoulders. Keep your body straight. Bring your upper body down

as close to the floor as possible. Do not allow chest or midsection to rest on the floor. Inhale down; exhale up. *Repetitions:* 5-15 times or as tolerated. (See Figure 4-8.)

Advanced—Men's Push-ups

Start in the same way as for the women's push-ups. As you do the exercise, though, keep your knees off the floor. *Repetitions:* 10-25 times or as tolerated. (See Figure 4-9.)

Figure 4-8. Women's Push-ups.

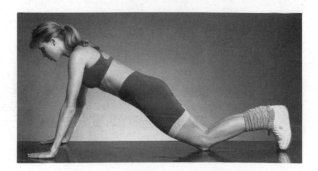

Figure 4-9. Men's Push-ups.

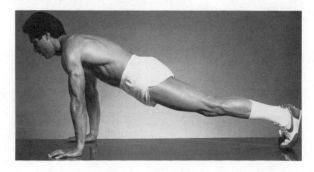

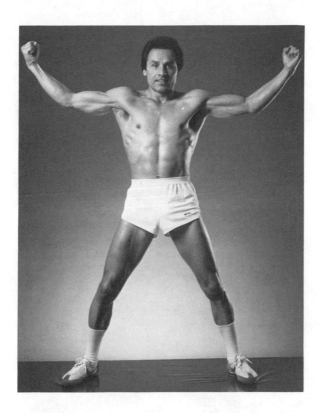

Figure 4-10.

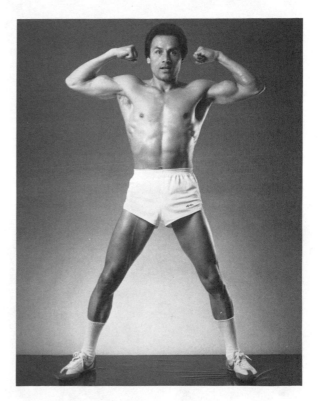

Figure 4-11. Lateral Arm Curls.

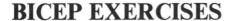
Figure 4-11. Lateral Arm Curls.

Figure 4-12. Standing Bicep Curls.

BICEP EXERCISES

Beginning—Lateral Arm Curls

Extend both arms out to your sides. As you bend them, contract the bicep (the front of the arm). Keep both legs slightly bent throughout the exercise. Light wrist weights would be excellent for this exercise. Exhale as the arms come in; inhale as they go out. *Repetitions:* 15-20 or as tolerated. (See Figures 4-10 and 4-11.)

Intermediate—Standing Bicep Curls

Select a barbell with a weight that is right for you. Grip the bar with an underhand grip or a reverse grip. Lock the elbows out at your side and bend both legs slightly. Drive the barbell up to the chest and slowly lower. Avoid inertial sway. Exhale on the way up; inhale on the way down. *Repetitions:* 10-15 or as tolerated. (See Figure 4-12.)

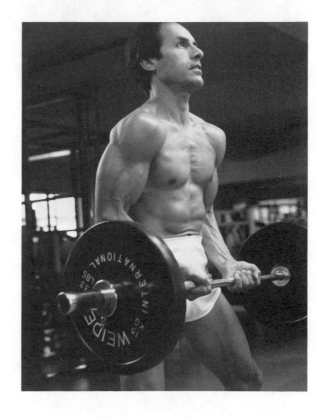

Advanced—Chin-ups

Hold onto a stable chinning bar with an underhand grip. Pull your weight up until your chin touches the bar. If you are unable to reach the bar, do quarter or half chin-ups or have someone assist you by holding on to your feet. Exhale on the way up; inhale on the way down. *Repetitions:* 5-15 times or as tolerated. (See Figure 4-13.)

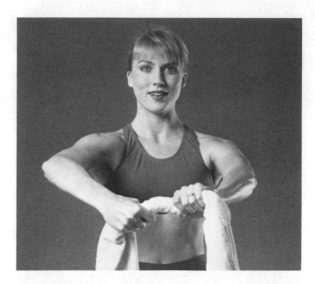

Figure 4-14. Wring the Towel Dry.

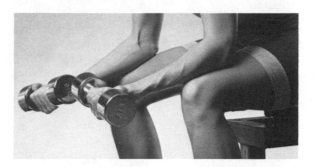

Figure 4-15.   **Figure 4-16. Seated Wrist Twist.**

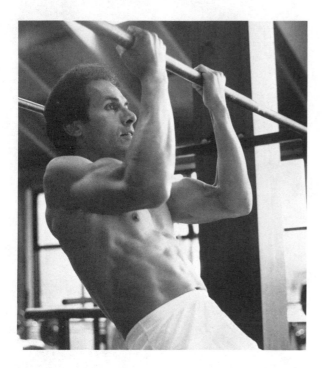

Figure 4-13. Chin-ups.

FOREARM EXERCISES

Beginning—Wring the Towel Dry

Take a dry towel, roll it up lengthwise, and wring it out. *Repetitions:* wring towel for 30 to 60 seconds. (See Figure 4-14.)

Intermediate—Seated Wrist Twist

Take a couple of light dumbbells and sit on a bench. Rest your forearms and elbows on your thighs. Start with palms facing upward. Twist the

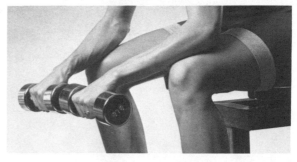

weights until they are facing down. Repeat back and forth. *Repetitions:* 15 or as tolerated. (See Figures 4-15 and 4-16.)

Advanced—Forearm Extensions and Forearm Flexions

Take a couple of light dumbbells and place your forearms on a flat surface with palms facing down. Allow the weight to drop below the forearms, then to raise above them. The second part (forearm flexions) is done virtually the same way with only two exceptions: (1) Begin with the palms facing up; allow the weight to drop all the way down to the fingertips, then lift above the forearms. (2) Generally, a little more weight can be used for forearm flexions than forearm extensions. *Repetitions:* 10-15 times or as tolerated. (See Figures 4-17 and 4-18.)

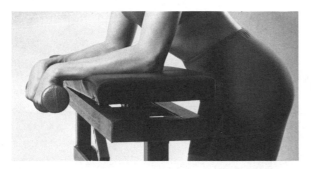

Figure 4-17.

Figure 4-18. Forearm Extensions and Forearm Flexions.

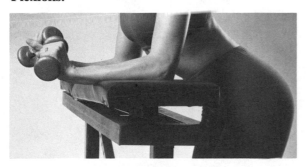

CHEST AND BUSTLINE EXERCISES

Beginning—Clap Four and Cross Four

Stand with both arms extended out in front of you. Bend both legs slightly. Clap hands 4 times and crossover 4 times. This exercise can also be done with light wrist weights. Clapping 4, crossing 4 constitutes one repetition. *Repetitions:* 15 times or as tolerated. (See Figures 4-19 and 4-20.)

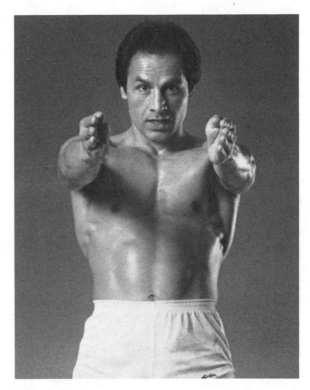

Figure 4-19.

Figure 4-20. Clap Four and Cross Four.

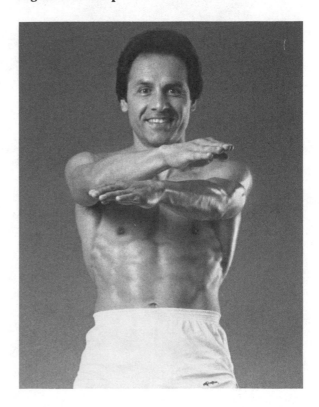

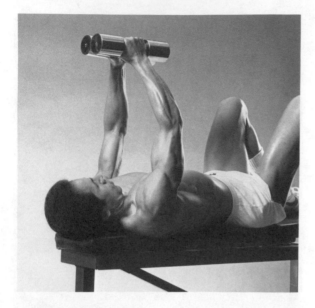

Figure 4-21.

Figure 4-22. Supine Laterals.

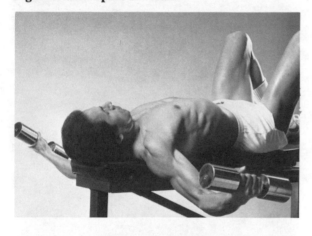

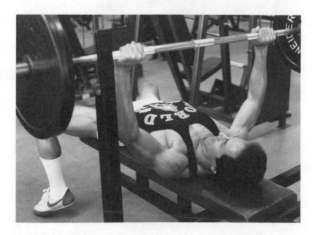

Figure 4-23. Bench Press.

Intermediate—Supine Laterals

Take a couple of light to moderate dumbbells and lie on a flat bench. Place both feet on the bench. Have palms facing each other. Keep both arms slightly bent. Open your arms laterally, allowing weights to drop to approximately shoulder level. Bring weights back up to starting position. Inhale on the way down; exhale on the way up. *Repetitions:* 10-15 times or as tolerated. (See Figures 4-21 and 4-22.)

Advanced—Bench Press

This exercise can be done with a barbell, dumbbells, Universal, Nautilus, Eagle Fitness Systems, and many other pieces of equipment. As depicted here, lie on your back on a flat bench. Grasp the barbell with a grip slightly wider than the shoulders. Bring the weight down to the chest in a controlled manner. Do not let the barbell bounce off your chest and keep your rear end glued to the bench. Return to starting position. Exhale on the way up; inhale on the way down. *Repetitions:* 10-15 times or as tolerated. (See Figure 4-23.)

UPPER BACK EXERCISES
(Avoid If You Have Back Problems)

Beginning—Reverse Shoulder Shrugs

Take a couple of light dumbbells. With the arms hanging straight, roll the shoulders up and back. Emphasize full range of motion. *Repetitions:* 15 times or as tolerated. (See Figure 4-24.)

Intermediate—Lat Pulldowns

This exercise can be done from either a seated or kneeling position. Grip overhead bar with a wide grip and pull down behind the head to your shoulders. Slowly return weight to starting

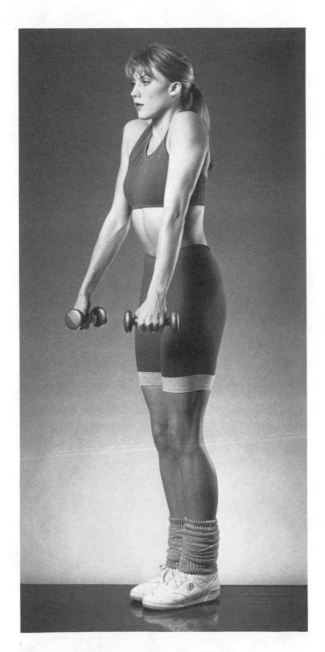

Figure 4-24. Reverse Shoulder Shrugs.

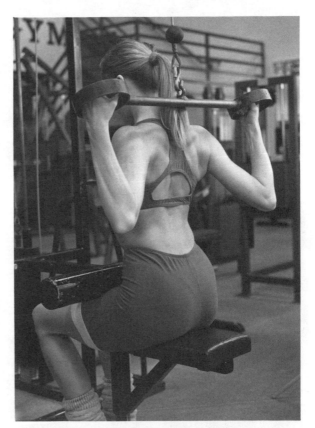

Figure 4-25. Lat Pulldowns.

Figure 4-26. Seated Rowing.

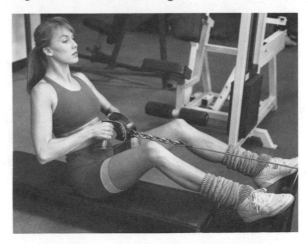

position. Keep your head forward so you don't bang your head with the bar. Exhale on the way down; inhale on the way up. *Repetitions:* 10-15 times or as tolerated. (See Figure 4-25.)

Advanced—Seated Rowing

Select correct weight. Starting position is seated with both knees bent, chest up, shoulders back, and head up. Lean forward and row back.

Bring rowing apparatus into the lower chest, upper abdominal region. Return weight to starting position slowly. *Discontinue this exercise if back pain ensues.* Exhale on inward motion. This exercise can also be done on a rowing machine or a Life Rower. *Repetitions:* 10-15 times or as tolerated. (See Figure 4-26.)

LOWER BACK EXERCISES
(Avoid If You Have Back Problems)

Beginning—Cat Back

On your hands and knees, relax your abdominals and let your back sag downward. Then tighten your abdominals and arch your back. Keep the movement smooth and controlled. Repeat. *Repetitions:* 10-15 times. (See Figure 4-27.)

Intermediate—Press-ups

Lie on your stomach and place your hands, palms down, at shoulder level. Gently raise the top half of your body, keeping the pelvis flat. Relax your pelvis, hips, and legs as you perform the exercise. Once you've gone up as far as you can, hold the position for 1 to 2 seconds and slowly lower yourself back down to the floor. Repeat. *Caution: discontinue if you experience back pain. Repetitions:* 10 times or as tolerated. (See Figure 4-28.)

Advanced—Back Extensions

Lie prone, hanging off the end of a back extension bench. Place your hands across your chest, on your temples, or clasped behind your head. Elevate your body until it is parallel to the floor. Return to starting position. Exhale on the way up; inhale down. *Caution: discontinue immediately if there is any back pain or discomfort. Repetitions:* 10-15 times or as tolerated. (See Figure 4-29.)

UPPER ABDOMINAL EXERCISES

Beginning—Quarter Sit-ups

Lie on your back with both knees bent. Extend both arms out in front of you. Lift head and shoulders a few inches off the ground and reach forward as far as you can. Stay up on the

Figure 4-27. Cat Back.

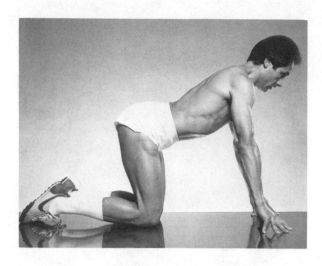

Figure 4-28. Press-ups.

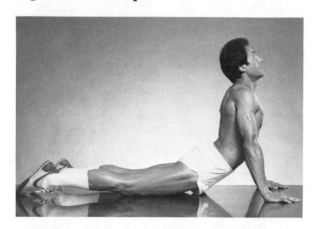

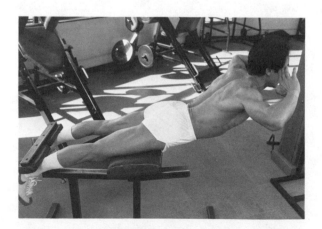

Figure 4-29. Back Extensions.

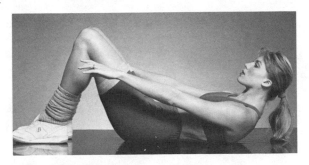

Figure 4-30. Quarter Sit-ups.

Figure 4-31. Three-Inch Sit-ups.

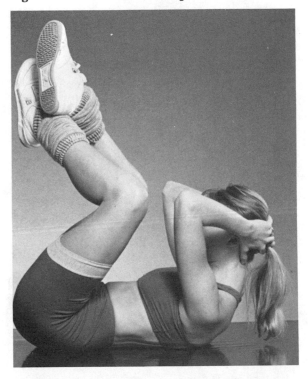

exercise, keeping the abdominals in a constant state of contraction. Middle and lower part of back remain on floor. Do not rest your head, shoulders, or abdominals until the exercise is completed. Exhale as you reach forward. *Repetitions:* 10-25 times or as tolerated. (See Figure 4-30.)

Intermediate—Three-Inch Sit-ups

Lie on your back, legs up and crossed. Clasp hands behind your head, but do not apply pressure to the back of the head. Lift the head and shoulders and bring both elbows to your knees. Maintain a 3-inch range of motion from elbows to knees. Exhale as elbows touch knees. *Optional:* hands may be placed on temples. *Repetitions:* 10-25 times or as tolerated. (See Figure 4-31.)

Advanced—Girl Scout Sit-ups

This is a four-part exercise. Lie on your back with one leg crossed over the other. Keep both feet off the floor. Place hands behind head, but do not put pressure on the head. Lift head and shoulders off the floor and perform exercise in the following sequence: (1) left elbow to right knee, 10 reps; (2) right elbow to right knee, 10 reps (cross legs in opposite direction); (3) right elbow to left knee, 10 reps; (4) left elbow to left knee, 10 reps.

Do not rest in between reps or leg changes. Exhale as elbow touches the knee. (See Figures 4-32 and 4-33.)

Figure 4-32.   **Figure 4-33. Girl Scout Sit-ups.**

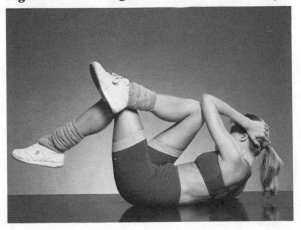

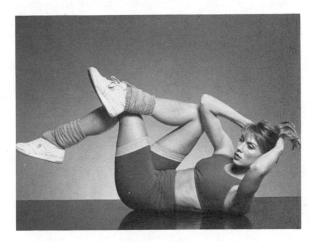

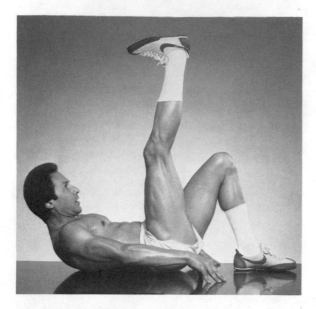

Figure 4-34. Single Leg Raise.

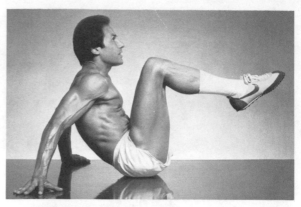

Figure 4-35. Knee Raise to Chest.

Figure 4-36. Highbar Leg Raises.

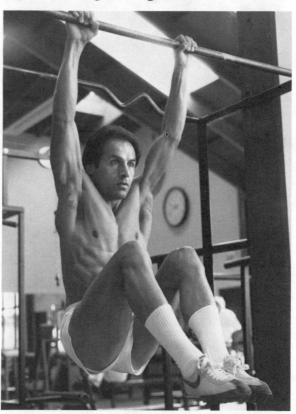

LOWER ABDOMINAL EXERCISES

Beginning—Single Leg Raise

Lie on your back, hands at your side, head up, and right foot dorsiflexed. Bend your left leg. Elevate right leg to 90 degrees. When returning right leg to starting position, do not let right foot touch the floor. Exhale as the leg comes up. Repeat exercise on opposite side. *Optional:* you may want to use light ankle weights for this exercise. If you want to work upper abdominals as well, lift head off the floor. *Repetitions:* 15-20 times or as tolerated. (See Figure 4-34.)

Intermediate—Knee Raise to Chest

From a seated position, extend both legs out in front of you and lean back on your arms. Tuck both knees into the chest and concentrate on keeping the abdominals contracted. Extend both legs as you return to starting position without resting the feet on the floor. Exhale as you tuck knees to chest. *Repetitions:* 10-25 times or as tolerated. (See Figure 4-35.)

Advanced—Highbar Leg Raises

Hang on a stable highbar. Lift both knees to about waist level with the legs bent. As you return legs to starting position, don't allow legs to drop all the way down. Avoid swinging during this exercise. Exhale as the legs come up; inhale down. *Repetitions:* 10-15 times or as tolerated. (See Figure 4-36.)

EXTERNAL OBLIQUE EXERCISES

Beginning—
Overhead Bent Arm Side Bends

From a standing position, feet about shoulder width, elevate both arms overhead and hold onto both elbows. Bend both knees slightly. Gently lean to the left, return to starting position, and then gently lean to the right. Exhale as you contract the obliques. Right/left constitutes one repetition. *Repetitions:* 15 times or as tolerated. (See Figure 4-37.)

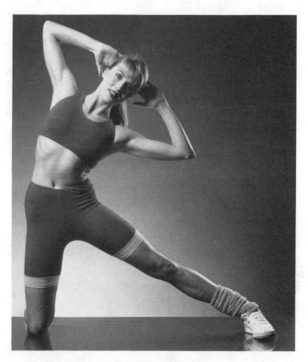

Figure 4-38. Kneeling Side Bends.

Intermediate—Kneeling Side Bends

Kneel on a soft surface. Extend left leg out to the side, foot flat and facing forward. Place hands behind head and gently lean to the left, contracting left side of waist. Keep left hip pushed forward throughout the exercise. Repeat on the opposite side. Exhale as you contract left oblique. *Repetitions:* 15-20 times or as tolerated. (See Figure 4-38.)

Advanced—
Standing Side Bends with Pulley

Using the bottom part of a cable pulley, select a light to moderate weight. Position yourself about 3 to 4 feet away. Hold onto cable pulley with right hand and place left hand behind head. Position feet wider than shoulders. Bend both knees slightly. Gently lean to your left, contracting left side of waist. Return to starting position. Exhale as you contract left oblique. Repeat on opposite side. *Repetitions:* 15 times or as tolerated. (See Figure 4-39.)

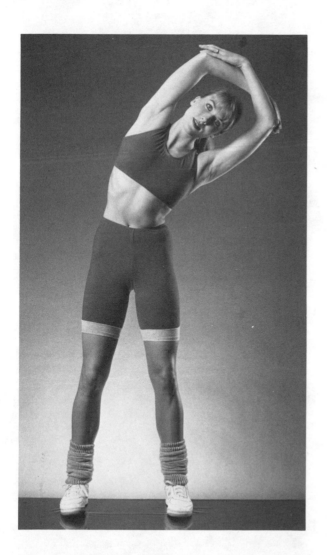

Figure 4-37. Overhead Bent Arm Side Bends.

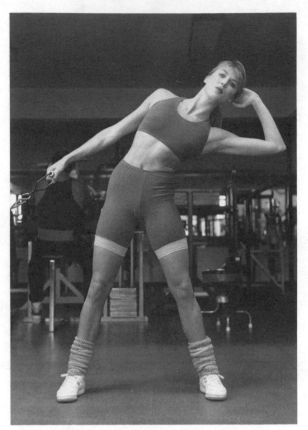

Figure 4-39. Standing Side Bends with Pulley.

HIP EXERCISES

Beginning—Supine Hip Raises

Lie on your back, knees bent and arms at your sides. Lift hips off the floor and contract your rear end. Lower hips, but do not allow them to touch the floor. Repeat. Exhale as you elevate hips. *Repetitions:* 15-25 times or as tolerated. (See Figure 4-40.)

Figure 4-40. Supine Hip Raises.

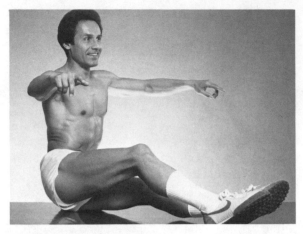

Figure 4-41. Hip Walk.

Intermediate—Hip Walk

Sit on the floor with both legs extended out in front of you. Elevate both arms and hip walk forward on a count of 10. Hip walk back for an equal count. *Repetitions:* 3-5 times or as tolerated. (See Figure 4-41.)

Advanced—Rear Leg Lifts

On your hands and knees, extend your right leg back until it is parallel to the floor. Bend both arms so weight is resting on forearms. Lower right foot to the floor, but don't let it touch, then return to parallel position. Keep right leg straight. *Discontinue if you experience back discomfort. Optional:* light ankle weights. Exhale as you lift right leg. *Repetitions:* 15-20 times or as tolerated. (See Figure 4-42.)

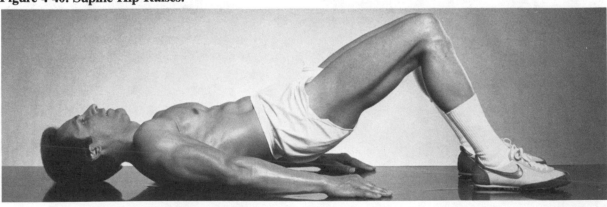

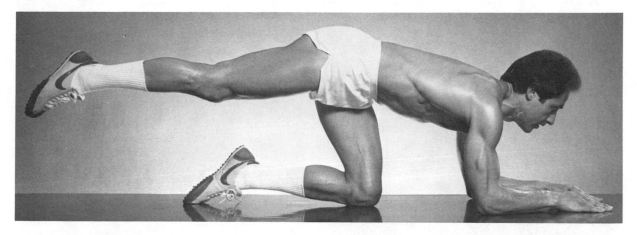

Figure 4-42. Rear Leg Lifts.

OUTER-THIGH EXERCISES

Beginning—Side Leg Raises

Lie on your right side and bend your right leg slightly. Straighten out left leg and keep left foot dorsiflexed and parallel to the ground. Tilt left hip forward. Elevate left leg and return to starting position, but do not let it touch or rest on right leg. Exhale as you lift leg. Repeat on opposite side. Optional: light ankle weights. *Repetitions:* 15-20 times or as tolerated. (See Figure 4-43.)

Figure 4-43. Side Leg Raises.

Intermediate—Standing Abductions

This exercise can be done with or without resistance. If working without resistance, hold onto a stable object, lock right leg, and dorsiflex right foot as you lift leg to the side. Stand on the ball of the left foot. Exhale as you lift the leg. If working with resistance, select a moderate weight and apply the same guidelines. Optional: light ankle weights. *Repetitions:* 15-20 times or as tolerated. (See Figure 4-44.)

Advanced—Seated Abductions

Seated on an abduction machine, select a weight that is appropriate for you. Open your legs as wide as possible and slowly return to starting

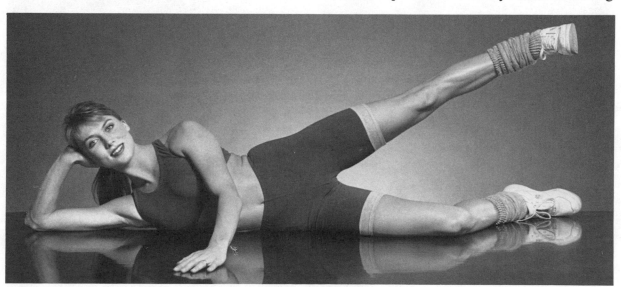

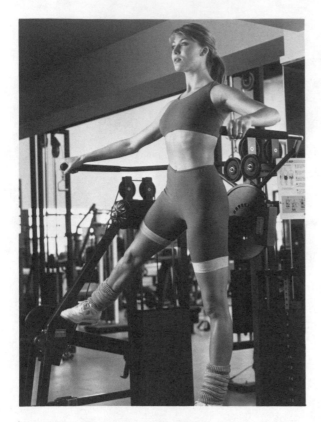

Figure 4-44. Standing Abductions.

Figure 4-45. Seated Abductions.

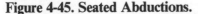

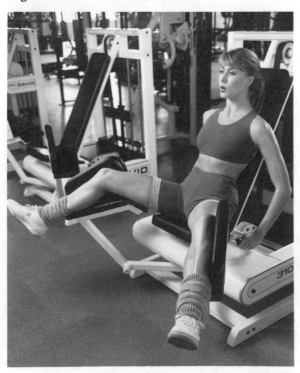

position. Use the 2-1-4 concept here. Open legs on a count of 2, hold for a count of 1, and return legs to starting position on a count of 4. Keep constant resistance on the outer thighs throughout exercise. Exhale as you open legs. *Repetitions:* 10-15 times or as tolerated. (See Figure 4-45.)

INNER-THIGH EXERCISES

Beginning— Ski Exercise with Knee Press

Start from a standing position with both feet and legs together. Bend both knees slightly. Move both legs laterally from side to side as though skiing. Simultaneously, press both knees against each other. Keep movement fluid and smooth. Repetitions: 15-20 times or as tolerated. (See Figure 4-46.)

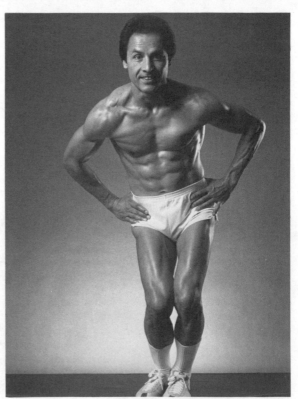

Figure 4-46. Ski Exercise with Knee Press.

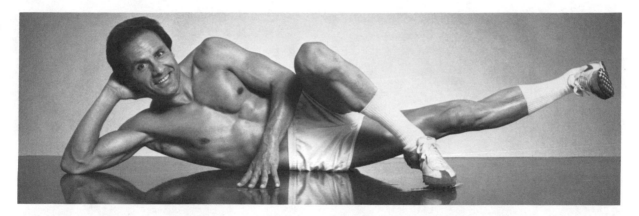

Figure 4-47. Inner Thigh Leg Raises.

Figure 4-48. Seated Adductions.

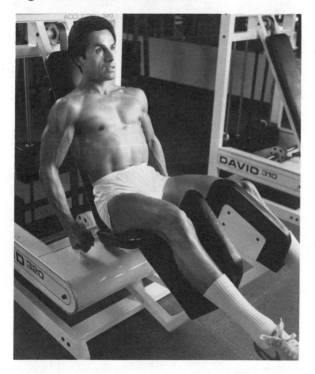

Advanced—Seated Adductions

Seated on an adduction machine, select a weight that is right for you. Open legs widely, push the weight in with both inner thighs, until they are together. Use the 2-1-4 concept. Close legs on a count of 2, hold for a 1 count, and open legs on a count of 4. Keep constant resistance on inner thighs throughout the exercise. Exhale as you bring legs together. *Repetitions:* 10-15 times or as tolerated. (See Figure 4-48.)

QUADRICEP EXERCISES

Beginning—Cycling

This exercise can be done on any bike ergometry. Adjust the seat so that leg on down pedal is bent about 5 to 10 degrees. No resistance should be applied during the first minute. Gradually work up to moderate resistance, keeping heart rate at approximately 70 percent of maximal heart rate. Start out with 5 minutes or as tolerated. Progressively work up to 15-20 minutes for aerobic benefits. (See Figure 4-49.)

Intermediate—Frontal Leg Raises

Hold onto a stable object. Place all your weight on your right leg. Extend left arm out to the side and lift your left leg from a locked position. Keep left foot dorsiflexed and stand on the ball of your right foot. Avoid inertia. *Optional:* light ankle weights. *Repetitions:* 15-20 times or as tolerated. (See Figure 4-50.)

Intermediate—
Inner Thigh Leg Raises

Lie on your right side. Bend left leg and place it in front of the right thigh. Dorsifex right foot, straighten out right leg, and lift off the floor. Exhale as you lift right leg. *Variation:* light ankle weights. *Repetitions:* 15-20 times or as tolerated. (See Figure 4-47.)

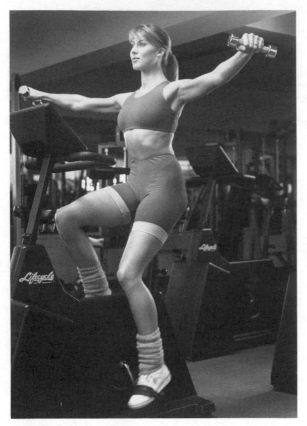

Figure 4-49. Cycling.

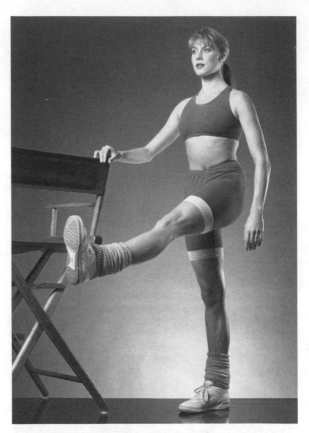

Figure 4-50. Frontal Leg Raises.

Figure 4-51. Leg Extensions.

Advanced—Leg Extensions

Select appropriate weight on leg extension machine. From a seated position, extend legs out to full extension. Limit range of motion to approximately 60 degrees. Feet can either be parallel to each other, turned in to work outer quads, or turned out to work inner quads. Lower weight slowly and controlled. Exhale as you extend legs. Repetitions: 10-15 or as tolerated. (See Figure 4-51.)

HAMSTRING EXERCISES

Beginning—Kneeling Hamstring Curls

Kneeling on your hands and feet, extend right leg out until it is parallel to floor. Bend right leg, bringing right heel as close to your hips as possible. Return to starting position. Perform this

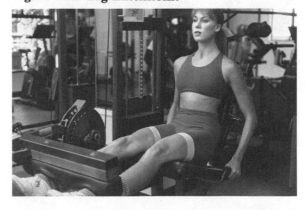

exercise slowly. Exhale as you bend right leg. *Repetitions:* 15-20 times or as tolerated. (See Figures 4-52 and 4-53.)

Intermediate—Cross-leg Curls

Lie on your stomach with your legs straight. Cross your right foot over your left. Next, try to bring the heel of the left foot to your hips with the right foot providing moderate resistance. Return

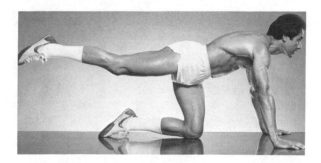

Figure 4-52.

Figure 4-53. Kneeling Hamstring Curls.

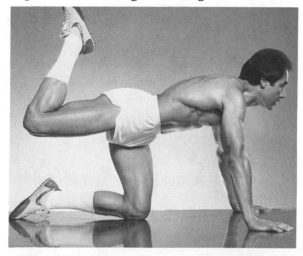

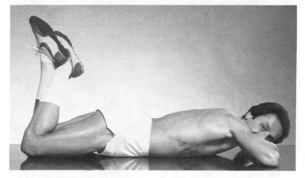

Figure 4-54. Cross-leg Curls.

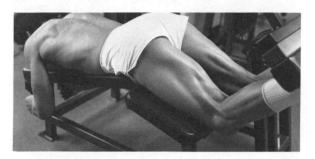

Figure 4-55. Leg Curls.

to starting position and repeat. Exhale as you're curling the leg. *Repetitions:* 10-15 times or as tolerated (See Figure 4-54.)

Advanced—Leg Curls

Select appropriate weight and lie on your stomach on a leg-curl machine. Position both knees slightly off the bench. Bring the heels as close to the rear end as possible, and slowly lower to starting position. Do not lift pelvis as you curl. *Avoid if you experience back discomfort.* Exhale on the curling motion. *Repetitions:* 10-15 or as tolerated. (See Figure 4-55.)

SHIN EXERCISES

Beginning—Seated Foot Flexion and Extension

Sit on the floor with both legs apart. Point the toes towards you, then point toes away from you. Concentrate on full range of motion for both exercises. Repetitions: 20 times each or as tolerated. (See Figure 4-56 and 4-57.)

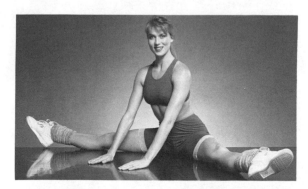

Figure 4-56.

Figure 4-57. Seated Foot Flexion and Extension.

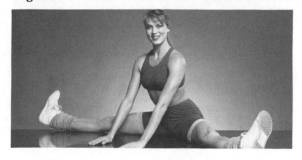

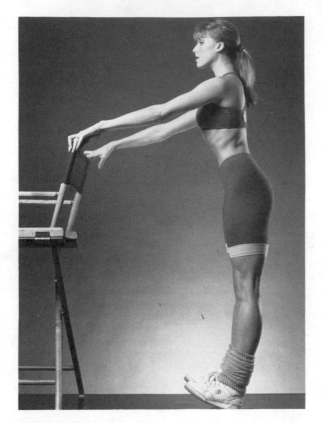

Figure 4-58. Toe Raises.

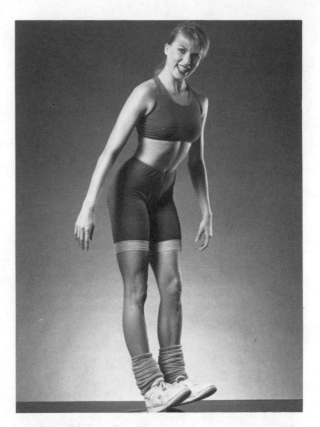

Figure 4-59. Heel Walk.

Intermediate—Toe Raises

Hold onto a chair and lift toes as high as possible off the floor. This exercise can also be done on a wooden or metal block for increased range of motion. *Repetitions:* 15-20 times or as tolerated. (See Figure 4-58.)

Advanced—Heel Walk

Walk on your heels forward and backward as tolerated. (See Figure 4-59.)

CALF EXERCISES

Beginning—Kneeling Calf Raises

From a kneeling position, bring your right leg forward. Position the knee directly above the toes. Place right forearm above right knee and apply pressure as you lift right heel. Repeat on opposite side. *Repetitions:* 15-20 times or as tolerated. (See Figure 4-60.)

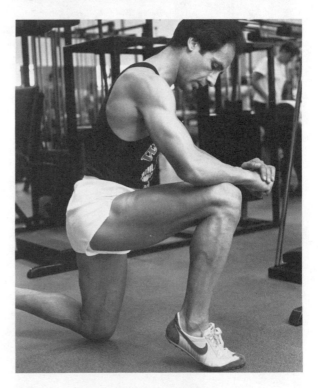

Figure 4-60. Kneeling Calf Raises.

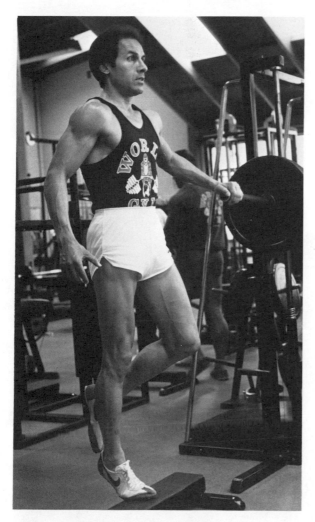

Figure 4-61. Single Leg Calf Raises.

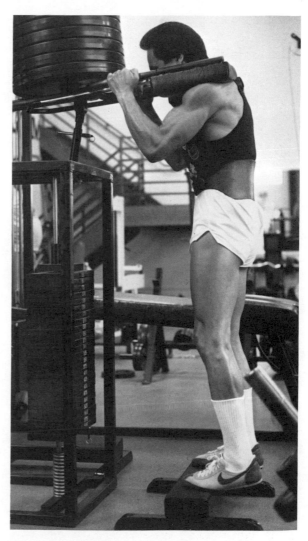

Figure 4-62. Bilateral Calf Raises.

Intermediate—
Single Leg Calf Raises

Hold onto a sturdy object. Place the ball of your right foot on a wooden or metal block or on the bottom step of a stairway. Lock your right leg and place left foot behind it. Lower right heel as far down as it will go, then lift as high as possible. Stretch both calves upon completion by letting both heels drop for about 30 seconds. *Repetitions:* 15 times or as tolerated. (See Figure 4-61.)

Advanced—Bilateral Calf Raises

This is a three-part exercise. Select an appropriate weight. Place the balls of both feet on a wooden or metal block. Feet may be positioned parallel, internally rotated, or externally rotated. Both legs should be straight. Drop and elevate both heels through the entire range of motion. Exhale as you lift. Stretch calves upon completion. *Repetitions:* 10-15 times or as tolerated. (See Figure 4-62.)

Chapter 5

TREATMENT AND PREVENTION OF BACK PROBLEMS

The success of back therapy should not be measured by the length of time it takes to become pain-free. It should be measured from a reduction in the incidence of recurrence.

—Robin McKenzie

Do you feel like you're "walking on eggshells" because of your back problems? Well, you're not alone. According to a recent United States Public Health Service report, there are somewhere in the vicinity of 70 million adults who have experienced at least one episode of severe and prolonged back pain.

It is generally agreed that backache is the second leading cause of pain in the U.S., second only to headaches. Back pain disrupts the lives of nearly eight out of every ten people. It often strikes at least twice, with 60 percent of those who recover from a lengthy attack of back pain being able to expect it to recur within a year. Most back pain episodes are temporary and subside with no treatment other than bed rest. Several recent studies have found that 80 to 90 percent of the people who suffer from this condition will return to work within two months, although more than half will suffer a serious recurrence.[1]

For the others who struggle for months and years with intractable, disabling back pain, the frequent absence of a definitive diagnosis can drive both patient and doctor to desperate lengths: (a) ill-advised surgery, often repeated; (b) acupuncture; (c) bitterness and cynicism about the medical establishment; (d) the seductiveness of depressants like Seconal, Demerol, Darvon, Valium, Codeine, Dalmane, and other such drugs; (e) depression, sometimes to the point of suicide.[2]

Fortunately, many back conditions can not only be treated successfully, but they could be prevented. The treatment in many cases is simple, effective, and inexpensive. In more serious conditions, the outcome may not be as favorable. Recovery, of course, depends on the extent of damage and proper therapeutic intervention. In a small percentage of cases, surgery may be necessary. However, it should only be as a last resort.

Another point to remember is that you continue doing the exercises after your back is healed. Continued correction of postural defects is equally important. These exercises should become a lifelong habit. As soon as most people get well, they stop their therapy altogether. In 90 percent of the cases, therapy or back exercises are resumed only when pain returns. *Your best bet against back pain is to maintain good flexibility, strengthen your back, maintain good postural alignment, and utilize proper lifting techniques.* Ten minutes minimum, 3 to 5 times per week, is all the back exercise that most of us need to do.

The primary focal point of this chapter will be on flexibility exercises for backs that are very tight and rigid. The secondary point of emphasis will be on maintaining normal range of motion. Anything other than that should be referred to a physician.

The following information is not only for those who have back problems now, but for those who also want to prevent them. Do keep in mind that many back problems require special medical attention. Therefore, do *not* self-diagnose. See a physician. Only he is prepared to evaluate and treat your condition in its entirety. The information provided in this text is to supplement or work in conjunction with your physician. If there is any conflict between what he says and what is written here, disregard what is written and follow his advice.

Basic Back Anatomy

The vertebral column consists of 33 vertebrae. There are 7 cervical, 12 thoracic, 5 lumbar, 5 sacral, and 4 coccygeal vertebrae. The vertebrae of the cervical, thoracic, and lumbar regions do not change throughout life; however, those of the sacral and coccygeal regions do. The 5 sacrals fuse, forming the sacrum, and the 4 coccygeal fuse to form the coccyx. On this basis, the adult has 26 vertebrae in the vertebral column.

The most stable region of the spine is the thoracic region. The least stable are the cervical, lumbar, and sacral regions. (See Figure 5-1.) This is one of the reasons why so many people have upper and lower back problems.

What Causes Back Problems?

The cause of back problems is by no means simple. If anything, it's quite complicated. Symptoms vary from short-term to chronic long-term pain and discomfort. Fortunately, most back problems are of short duration, while others have the capacity to cripple. The following are some of the more common causes of back problems:

1. Poor posture[3]
2. Traumatic injury
3. Obesity and weak abdominal muscles[4]
4. Poor muscle tone
5. Congenital conditions
6. Emotional stress and tension[5]
7. Rheumatoid arthritis and osteoarthritis

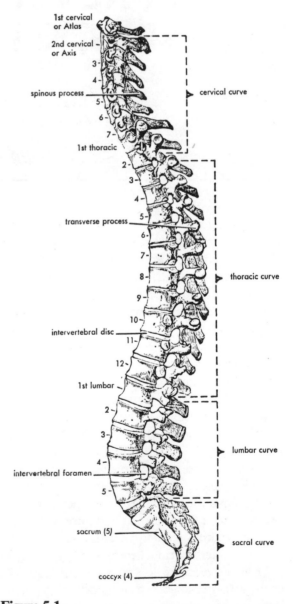

1st cervical or Atlas
2nd cervical or Axis
3-
4-
spinous process
5-
6-
7-
1st thoracic
2-
3-
4-
transverse process
5-
6-
7-
8-
9-
10-
intervertebral disc
11-
12-
1st lumbar
2-
3-
4-
intervertebral foramen
5-
sacrum (5)
coccyx (4)

cervical curve
thoracic curve
lumbar curve
sacral curve

Figure 5-1.

8. Sedentary lifestyles, which lead to a loss of spinal flexibility
9. Bending forward too much during the course of the day

The following conditions also contribute to bad backs, but generally not as frequently: (a) leg length discrepancies; (b) osteoporosis (fragile and brittle bones); (c) benign and malignant tumors; (d) osteoarthritis with degenerative discs.

The most common causes of recurrent lower back problems, in athletes and non-athletes alike, are: not allowing sufficient time for the injured part to heal and lack of appropriate rehabilitation before return to the pretrauma level of physical activity.[6]

Many back problems are caused by loss of lordosis (curvature in the lower back), according to Robin McKenzie. Loss of lordosis, very simply, is keeping your lower back rounded instead of arched. McKenzie's research has shown that, when the back is rounded or stooped for a prolonged period of time, it will generally produce low back pain. Some of the activities that frequently produce back pain when lordosis is not maintained are:

1. Prolonged sitting with the back rounded and shoulders slumped. This can be avoided by sitting up and placing a small lumbar roll between the chair and your lower back. Interrupt the frequency of flexion (bending forward) by getting up occasionally and bending your back backwards 5 to 10 times.[7]

2. Prolonged bending such as vacuuming, ironing, or gardening. This can be alleviated by keeping the back in a more upright position and intermittently bending backwards.[8]

3. Incorrect lifting. Even though you've heard it many times, the probability of having back pain or back problems increases considerably with improper lifting. Keep your back straight and lift with your legs, not your back.

According to Robin McKenzie, a physical therapist and author of *Treat Your Own Back* and *The Lumbar Spine—Mechanical Diagnosis and Therapy,* many people think that lower back pain is caused by strained muscles. This is seldom the case. The cause of nearly all simple mechanical lower back pain lies in the discs between the vertebrae and in the tissues surrounding them.[9]

Hundreds of thousands of people suffer needlessly from back pain every day. The primary reason for this, according to McKenzie, is a lack of awareness, neglect, and back mismanagement. When in acute pain, we are usually unable to think clearly about our trouble and simply seek relief from the pain. On the other hand, when we have recovered from an acute episode, most of us quickly forget about our lower back problems.

One final note: The success of back therapy should not be measured by the length of time it takes to become pain-free. It should be measured from a reduction in the incidence of recurrence.

WHAT IS LORDOSIS?

Lordosis is the sway or hollow of the lower back. The condition is not an abnormal one, as many have been led to believe. Nearly everyone has a slight hollow or sway on the back. What is abnormal is a pronounced increase or decrease of degrees in the hollow or sway of the lower back.

Causes of Lordosis

A pronounced lordosis (swayback) may occur at birth or later in life. This condition may also be attributed to the following:

1. Obesity (body weight 15 percent or greater above ideal weight)
2. Weak lower back muscles
3. Weak abdominal muscles
4. Wearing high-heeled shoes

Unfortunately, there are still some people in the medical profession and some physical educators who continue to advocate the avoidance of all extension exercises (bending backwards). They fear that bending backwards will weaken the lower back and deepen the inward curve of the spine. Dr. Robert Martin of Pasadena, California, and designer of the Gravity Guiding System, feels that the exact opposite is true. Dr. Martin points out that "complete extension will not cause lordosis. The fact that most of those with lordosis have never practiced extension to any serious degree, and yet have such prevalent postural fault, gives us proof that completely extending the spine does not cause lordosis."

To straighten, lengthen, and correctively condition the spine is to use the "rule of all joints," that is, to employ maximum mobility. Orthopedics dictates that complete mobility of a joint is a necessity for joint health and that no joint is excluded. For joint health, every joint must be taken through its full range of motion. The joints of the spine are no exception to this rule of orthopedics. For the spine to gain its maximum mobility, it must be trained and developed in both complete extension and complete flexion. When the spine is then allowed to relax in the erect posture, the supporting and influencing structures will take the most neutral position between the two extremes of complete extension and complete flexion.[10]

Treatment for Pronounced Lordosis

1. Decrease weight, if overweight or obese.
2. Strengthen upper and lower abdominal muscles.
3. Maintain good posture.
4. Complete flexion and complete extension unless contraindicated by your physician or physical therapist.
5. Shorten hamstrings to tilt the pelvis in a posterior direction. This can be done with any type of leg flexion exercise, such as leg-curls. However, if any type of leg flexion exercise bothers the back, it should be discontinued.

WHAT IS KYPHOSIS?

Kyphosis (humpback) is an abnormal, outward curvature of the spine. Humpbacks, in varying degrees, are frequently seen in the elderly.

Causes of Kyphosis

The following are a few of the causes of kyphosis:

1. Poor posture resulting from insufficient support by the upper back muscles and the constant downward pull of gravity.
2. Tuberculosis in one or more of the vertebral bodies. Although rare today, the bodies could be diseased, weakened, even eaten away, then crushed by the weight of the body.[11]
3. Muscular imbalance.
4. Osteoporosis.[12]
5. Fracture.
6. Metabolic diseases.
7. Tumor.
8. Congenital anomaly (irregularity at birth).
9. Ankylosing spondylitis, also known as "bamboo spine."

Treatment for Kyphosis

Depending on whether it's structural or functional, some forms of kyphosis can be treated with:

1. Correction of posture
2. Extension type exercises
3. Strengthening exercises

SCOLIOSIS

Scoliosis is a lateral curvature or convexity of the spine. It usually consists of two curves, the original one and a compensatory curve in the opposite direction. Scoliosis can generally be broken down into two categories: (a) functional scoliosis and (b) structural scoliosis. Functional scoliosis can be corrected; structural scoliosis, except for surgery, generally cannot be corrected. (See Figure 5-3.)

Causes of Scoliosis

Scoliosis may result from chronic or acute lumbar sacral sprain, defective development of

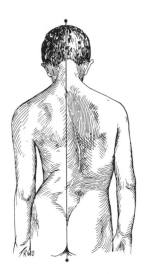

Figure 5-2.

the spine (congenital scoliosis), habitual standing or sitting in an improper position (habit scoliosis), vertebral or spinal disease (osteopathic scoliosis), rickets (rachitic scoliosis), weakened spinal muscles (myopathic scoliosis), rheumatism of the dorsal muscles (rheumatic scoliosis), and an inequality in the length of the two legs (static scoliosis), resulting from either a fracture or congenital deformity of a lower extremity.[13]

Treatment for Scoliosis

Due to the complexity of this condition, it is advised that you check with your physician for medical guidelines.

TREATMENT OF CERVICAL (UPPER BACK) STRAIN

Treatment for Acute Cervical Strain

1. Absolute bed rest
2. Stretching exercises prescribed by your physical therapist
3. McKenzie cervical therapy
4. Ice
5. Firm mattress preferable
6. Cervical collar

7. McKenzie cervical roll (provides support and reduces strain to the cervical spine while sleeping)
8. Massage
9. Anti-inflammatory medication if prescribed by physician
10. Cervical traction
11. Avoiding movements that increase the symptoms
12. No strengthening exercises

Treatment For Chronic and Prophylactic (Preventive) Cervical Strain

1. Correction of posture
2. Warm baths or whirlpool
3. McKenzie cervical roll
4. Stretching exercises prescribed by your physical therapist
5. Range of motion exercises prescribed by your physical therapist
6. Firm mattress preferable
7. Appropriate activities compatible with age and physical condition

TREATMENT OF LUMBAR (LOWER BACK) STRAIN

Treatment for Acute Lumbar Strain

1. Absolute bed rest
2. McKenzie lumbar therapy
3. Lower back stretches prescribed by your physician or physical therapist
4. Ice
5. Firm mattress, bed-board, or waterbed (whichever provides the greatest relief)
6. McKenzie lumbar roll
7. Massage
8. Anti-inflammatory medication, if prescribed by a physician
9. Lumbar traction
10. Avoid movements or positions that increase symptoms
11. No strengthening exercises

Treatment For Chronic and Prophylactic (Preventive) Lumbar Strain

1. Reduction of weight
2. Correction of posture
3. McKenzie lumbar roll
4. Warm baths or whirlpool
5. Firm mattress, bed-board, or waterbed (whichever provides the greatest relief)
6. Lower back stretches prescribed by your physical therapist
7. Appropriate activities compatible with age and physical condition

DO'S AND DON'TS OF GOOD BODY MECHANICS

The use of good body mechanics is essential for the effective treatment of back dysfunction and derangement. The following are a few examples:

Do keep your weight under control.

Do stand tall, keeping the back straight and maintaining lordosis.

Do strengthen your back with the right exercises *but not during the acute stage.*

Do develop and use both sides of the body equally.

Do bend the knees and keep the back flat when lifting objects.

Do turn and face any object you're lifting.

Do sit correctly, and interrupt prolonged sitting at regular intervals by standing up, walking around, or stretching backwards.

Do sit in a fairly sturdy chair with a straight back. If seated for a prolonged period of time, use a lumbar roll.

Do be aware of your posture at all times.

Don't permit yourself to become overweight or obese.

Don't allow your back to become weak and atrophied.

Don't stoop or slouch.

Don't lift with your legs straight.

Don't lift a heavy object higher than your waist.

Don't stand or sit too long in any one position.

Don't sit with a rounded back.

Don't walk with a rounded back.

Don't sit in a soft chair or a deep couch.

Don't let the force of gravity pull you down. It's not only bad for you, but it makes you look older.

Don't overload or carry unbalanced loads.

Don't let your abdominal muscles get flabby. Avoid "spare tires."

Don't do any of the exercises if your symptoms are worse during or immediately after exercising or if they become worse the next day.

Don't use high-heeled shoes.

ULTIMATE FITNESS BACK STRETCHES AND EXERCISES

Seated Low Back Stretch

Sit on a chair. Slowly bend over and reach down for your ankles. Relax. Hold this position for 30 seconds or count to 10 very slowly. Uncurl slowly into an upright position, using your arms

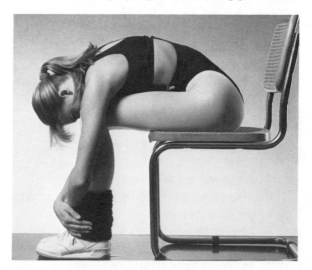

Figure 5-4. Seated Low Back Stretch.

to assist you and raising your head last. *Frequency:* intermittently during the day as needed. (See Figure 5-4.)

Low Back Stretch

Sit with feet together, legs extended in front of you. Keep both feet pointed toward you. Slowly bend forward, holding onto your knees, calves, ankles, or feet. Gently pull forehead toward knees. Do not bounce and don't hold your breath. Hold for approximately 30 seconds. Slowly return to starting position. *Frequency:* once per day or as prescribed by physician or physical therapist. (See Figure 5-5.)

Single Knee to Chest

Lie flat on your back with both knees bent. Bring right knee up and pull it firmly to the chest with both hands. Keep right foot dorsiflexed. Hold for 30 seconds, and return to starting position. Switch to opposite side. *Frequency:* once per day. (See Figure 5-6.)

Double Knee to Chest

Lie on your back, arms at the side, knees bent. Bring both knees up and pull them firmly to the chest with both hands. Hold for approximately 30 seconds. It is important that you do not straighten your knees as you lower your legs. *Frequency:* once per day. (See Figure 5-7.)

Knee Over

Lie flat on your back with legs straight and arms extended out to the side. Place right hand on the outer part of the left knee and gently pull it across the body. Bring bent knee as close to the floor as possible. If the bent knee is up close to the chest, it will stretch the middle and lower back. If the bent knee is below the hips, it will stretch the lower back. Keep both shoulders grounded or flat on the floor and the right leg extended. Return to center and repeat on opposite side. Hold stretch for 30 seconds on each side. *Frequency:* once per day. (See Figure 5-8.)

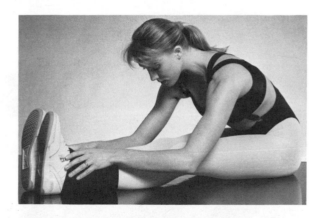

Figure 5-5. Low Back Stretch.

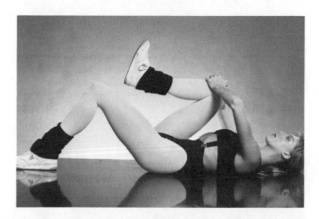

Figure 5-6. Single Knee to Chest.

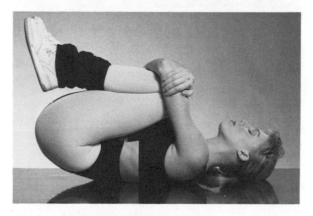

Figure 5-7. Double Knee to Chest.

Prone Lying

Lie face down on a comfortable surface with your arms beside your body and your head turned to the side. Take a few deep breaths and

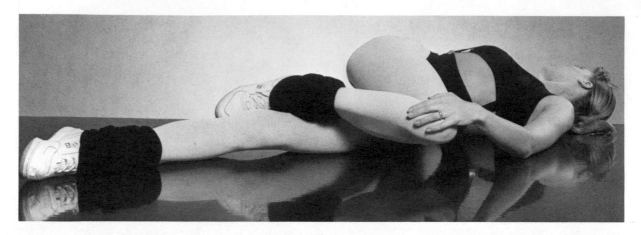

Figure 5-8. Knee Over.

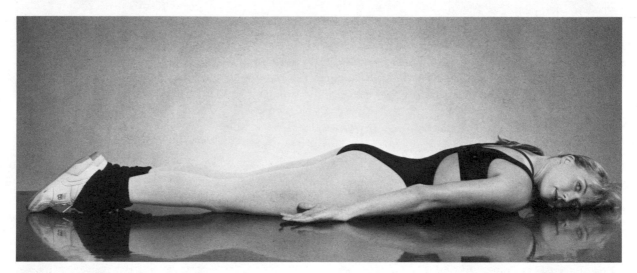

Figure 5-9. Prone Lying.

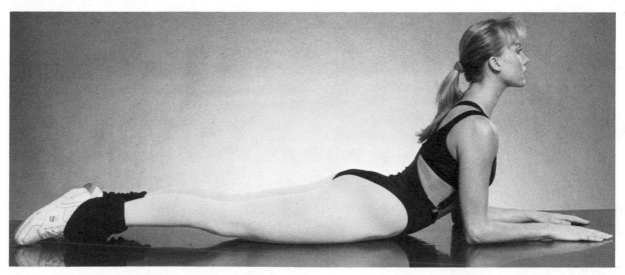

Figure 5-10. Half Press-ups.

relax completely for approximately 2 to 3 minutes. *Frequency:* once per day. (See Figure 5-9.)

Half Press-ups

Lie face down on a rug or exercise mat. Allow your lower back to relax completely. Come halfway up and place your weight on your elbows and forearms. Hold this position for approximately 1 minute and return to starting position. Rest for 30 seconds before coming back up again. Avoid if there is pain or discomfort to lower back. *Repetitions:* up 3 times, resting weight on elbows for 1 minute duration each time. *Frequency:* once per day. (See Figure 5-10.)

Three-Quarter or Full Press-ups

Lie face down on a soft surface. Place your hands, palms down, at shoulder level and raise the top half of your body, keeping the pelvis flat. It is important that you relax your pelvis, hips, and legs as you perform this exercise. Once you have maintained this position for a second or two, lower yourself back to the starting position and repeat. Exhale on the way up. Inhale on the way down. Avoid if you experience lower back

pain or discomfort. *Repetitions:* 10 times or as tolerated. *Frequency:* once per day or as directed by a physician or physical therapist. (See Figure 5-11.)

Standing Backbends

Stand straight with your feet slightly apart. Place your hands in the small of the back. Bend backwards from the waist as far as you can, using your hands as a fulcrum. Keep both legs as straight as possible. Once you have held the position for a second, return to starting position and repeat. If you get dizzy when you lean back, hold on to a firm object with one hand. *Repetitions:* 10 times. *Frequency:* intermittently during the day, particularly after sustained back flexion. (See Figure 5-12.)

SLEEPING POSITIONS: A CAUSE OF BACK PAIN

Pain experienced during sleep is not uncommon. Robin McKenzie points out that this causes considerable distress when it interferes

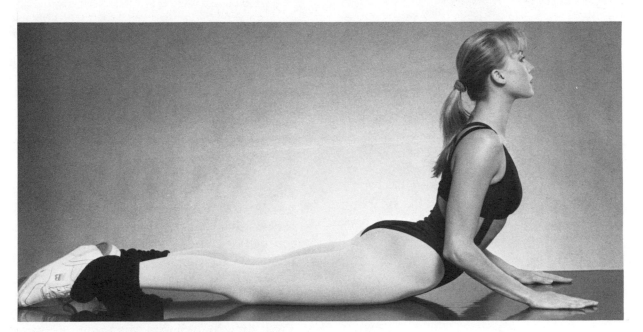

Figure 5-11. Three-Quarter or Full Press-ups.

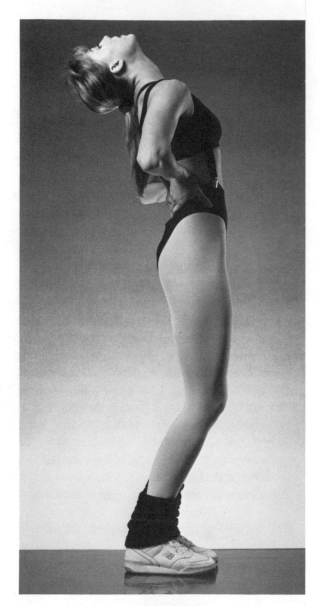

Figure 5-12. Standing Backbends.

sleep is difficult to influence.

2. The surface on which one is lying. For the majority of people the mattress itself should not be too hard, whereas the base on which the mattress rests must be firm and unyielding. This allows adequate support for the contours of the body without placing stresses on the spine. Usually, the surface on which one is lying is easily corrected or modified.

When dealing with pain produced lying in bed, McKenzie makes these recommendations:

> Because of the natural contours of the body—wider at the shoulders and pelvis than at the waist—and due to the lordotic curvature of the lower back, the lumbar area may be placed under stress in the: (a) prone position (lying on stomach); (b) supine position (lying on back); (c) side lying position.
>
> This is particularly so when a hard mattress is supported by a firm and unyielding base. If this is thought to be the cause of the problem, the patient should use a lumbar-support roll. When lying prone, the roll will prevent extreme extension in the lumbar spine (lower back). When lying supine (on back), with the legs outstretched, the roll will fill the gap between the lower back and the mattress and prevent sagging of the spine into flexion. When lying on the side, it will fill the gap between the pelvis and ribs and prevent sagging of the spine into flexion. This type of lumbar support in bed usually works quickly or not at all, and should be tried for about three nights.[15]

A beach towel folded end-to-end and then rolled crosswise usually fits around the average middle. If this is too big, a bath towel folded lengthwise can be used instead. Each patient will have to experiment to find the correct size of the lumbar roll required in each particular case. The towel should be wrapped around the belt line and the two ends attached together. If left loose, the roll will not remain in place and may, when positioned anywhere else other than at the waist, further increase the stresses placed on the spine.[16]

Another option is to purchase the McKenzie Night Roll from Orthopedic Physical Therapy Products in Minneapolis, Minnesota.

When the base of the mattress is not firm

with sleep patterns over a long period of time, and it requires attention when the patient regularly wakes up with pain in the morning, the pain often abating as the day progresses.

There are two factors to be investigated:[14]

1. The lying posture itself. This is different for each person and must be dealt with individually. The lying posture during

enough or the mattress itself is too soft, stresses may also be placed on the lower back. Because of the costs involved in replacing a mattress or its base, an alternative to buying a new one is to try placing the mattress on the floor to achieve a firm, flat base. If there is no improvement after sleeping three or four nights on a flat surface, it is unlikely that this is the answer to the patient's problem.[17]

There is a small number of people who require a less firm mattress. This mattress could easily be created by placing pillows at both ends of the bed in between the mattress and its base to form a "dish" shape.[18]

It is also recommended that you use a pillow that fits the space between your head and the mattress, so that your head is in line with your spine—tilted neither down nor up.

If uncertain, check with either your physician or physical therapist to determine which sleeping positions are most appropriate for your back condition.

RECOMMENDED AND NON-RECOMMENDED PHYSICAL ACTIVITIES FOR THOSE WITH BACK PROBLEMS

The following recommended and non-recommended physical activities are offered as a general guide to anyone suffering from a back problem. For specific guidelines, it is recommended that you check with your physician before undertaking any activity.

Recommended Physical Activities

1. Progressive walking: (a) watch your posture; (b) maintain lordosis; (c) avoid the "looking for dimes syndrome" (looking down at the ground as you're walking); (d) wear a comfortable pair of jogging shoes (no high-heeled shoes).
2. Cycling: (a) preferably stationary; (b) initially, 5-10 minutes or as tolerated; (c) in general, keep exercise heart rate between 120-150 BPM, or at 70 percent of maximal heart rate. See the chart on page 30; (d) cycle at a moderate pace with moderate resistance; (e) elevate seat to get good leg extension; (f) don't slouch; sit upright; (g) avoid bikes with low handle bars; (h) if sitting aggravates back pain, discontinue cycling.
3. Stretching: (a) refer to Chapter 2 for stretching exercises; (b) stretch a minimum of 10 minutes or as tolerated; (c) static stretching only; (d) hold each stretch for about 30 seconds; (e) maintain rhythmic breathing; (f) stretch within your limits and listen to your body; (g) there should be no pain associated with stretching.
4. Swimming: (a) the duration should be about 5 to 10 minutes initially or as tolerated; (b) swimming works every muscle in the body while developing the cardiovascular system; (c) emphasize endurance swimming over sprinting; (d) use overhand crawl, breast stroke, or side strokes; avoid back stroke and the butterfly; (e) if you have a cervical (upper back) problem, use a snorkel to avoid turning the head from side to side.

Non-Recommended Physical Activities

All back problems are individualized and should be diagnosed and treated by a qualified physician. Any attempt to self-diagnose is not recommended. The information provided here is to make you aware of exercises that may be potentially damaging to your back.

If you have a back problem or are experiencing back pain or discomfort, the following activities should generally be avoided due to sudden falls, rough contact, sudden impact, unusual twisting, and direct stress or pressure on the back. When your back is fully healed, resumption of any of these activities will depend on your physician or physical therapist.

Non-Recommended Physical Activities

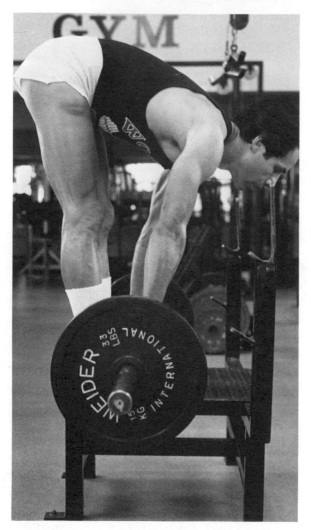

Deadlifts.

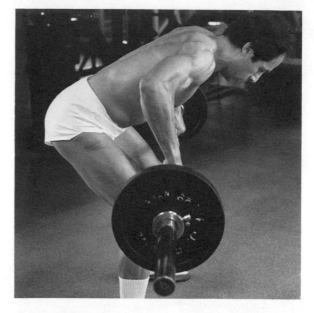

Bentover Rowing.

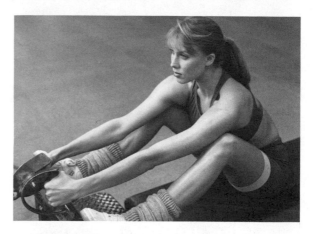

Seated Rowing.

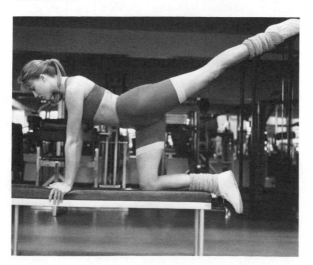

Rear Leg Lifts.

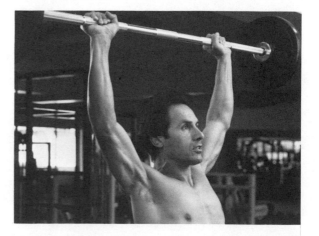

Military Press.

AVOID THESE EXERCISES IF YOU HAVE A BACK PROBLEM

1. Aerobic classes (high and low impact)
2. Back-packing
3. Baseball
4. Basketball
5. Bowling
6. Deadlifts
7. Football
8. Golf
9. Gymnastics
10. Handball
11. Horseback riding
12. Ice skating
13. Ice hockey
14. Jogging/Running
15. Karate
16. Leg-curls
17. Liferower (rowing machine)
18. Military presses (overhead presses)
19. Nautilus back extension, rotary torso, seated rowing, and hip-extension machines
20. Nordic Skier (cross country skiing machine)
21. Plow stretch
22. Prone hyperextensions
23. Racquetball
24. Roller skating
25. Rope-jumping
26. Side bends
27. Side leg raises
28. Sit-ups
29. Snow and water skiing
30. Soccer
31. Squats with weights on shoulders
32. Stairmaster
33. Standing or seated waist twist
34. Standing toe touches
35. Straight leg raises
36. Straight leg standing bentovers (A.K.A. "Good morning" exercise)
37. Tennis
38. Upright rowing
39. Versaclimber
40. Volleyball   41. Walking in high heels

QUESTIONS AND ANSWERS ABOUT BACK INJURIES

What is a Ruptured or Herniated Disc?

A ruptured or herniated disc is a spinal condition in which the jelly-like inner pulp of the disc, called "nucleus pulposus," ruptures as a result of too much pressure. Ruptured discs generally occur from incorrect lifting, falls, and auto accidents. In some cases, it can be from something as simple as bending over to open a drawer or turning to answer a phone call.

While working at the Beverly Hills Health Club in the early seventies, I came across a man in his late twenties, who told me an interesting story about a serious back accident he had. The man was traveling through Texas, and he walked into a public restroom that apparently had an old toilet seat with rust and corroded bolts supporting it. As the man was sitting on the toilet seat, one of the bolts snapped loose, and the seat dropped about a half an inch on one side. One of the discs in his lower back ruptured, and he has since required two major back surgeries. I also had a friend who reached up to take something off a shelf, when suddenly he felt something "snap" in the back of his neck. A few months later, he also had spinal surgery after a myelogram revealed a ruptured cervical disc.

What does all this information tell us? The message is clear. No one is immune to back injury. Never take anything for granted. We're all vulnerable. So work on your back. Maintain good posture, sufficient strength, and adequate flexibility. Last year, there were more than two-hundred thousand patients who underwent laminectomies (disc surgery). I'm sure none of them ever expected to see the day when they would be wheeled into the operating room for back surgery.

Ruptures can occur in any of the spinal vertebrae, but the area that is affected most often is the lower back. A rupture looks like an old basketball whose outer layer has split open, allowing the dark inner tubing to bulge out. The bulging dark inner tubing is similar to the ruptured jelly-like substance in the disc. What happens is that this bulge may begin to put pressure on the nerve or nerve roots and possibly cause neurological (nerve) inflammation. The inflamed nerve may then cause the muscles supplied by that nerve to spasm, making movement not only difficult but painful. In many cases, the pain and possible numbness will radiate into the upper or lower extremities. Those who suffer sciatica, for example, are very familiar with the symptoms I'm describing.

Is "Popping" Your Back Bad for You?

According to Dr. Michael Schiffman, orthopedic surgeon at Centinela Hospital Medical Center in Los Angeles, "the practice in and of itself, is not harmful." Dr. Schiffman explains that, "the popping sound is caused by the distraction of a joint that creates negative pressure on the synovial fluid contents. This negative pressure produced within a closed joint space causes the precipitation of gas bubbles, which produce the popping sound when formed." The same thing occurs when you "pop" or "crack" your knuckles.

If you are popping your back to relieve existing back pain, discard the self-manipulation and consult your physician.

Can a Vertebral Disc "Slip" Out of Place?

The entire disc cannot slip, since the outer casing is tightly anchored to the vertebral bodies above and below, but the side of the casing can weaken, and that can mean trouble. The center of the disc is under pressure, and a weakened sidewall may bulge, just like an automobile tire. Sometimes this could even tear completely and permit the inner material of the disc to escape. [19]

Can Pain and a Numb Tingling Sensation in the Leg be Indicative of a Lower Back Problem?

It most definitely can. With many people, the problem of origin might very well be the lower back. A ruptured disc is a good example of this. However, there might be other causes, which should be examined. Conditions such as poor or restricted circulation in the legs (intermittent claudication) or any condition directly involving injury or damage to the nerves or nerve roots should not be overlooked.

If you are experiencing numbness and pain in the lower extremities, do not attempt self-diagnosis or self-treatment. Have your physician examine you and let him or her make the appropriate diagnosis and recommendations.

Do You Recommend Waterbeds for People with Back Problems?

That depends on the individual and the extent of the back condition. A waterbed might not necessarily be the best or most beneficial sleeping surface for someone suffering from back pain. In some cases they're good, and in others they're not. The response is not always linear. Generally, the recommendation is to sleep on a firm mattress. However, if someone is having problems sleeping on a hard bed and switches over to a waterbed, and the symptoms either improve or disappear, then use a waterbed. Barbara Stone, of the South Bay Spine Center in Los Angeles, points out that how you are first thing in the morning is also indicative of the "right or wrong" sleeping surface. My recommendation is to sleep on a surface that provides you with the greatest amount of relief, the least amount of irritation, and the best sleep you can get.

Do You Recommend a Lumbar Roll for People with Back Problems?

A lumbar roll is a small, rounded cushion, which fits snugly between your lower back and a chair or car seat. Its primary purpose is to maintain a slight hollow or sway in the lower back, especially while sitting for lengthy periods of time. If you have poor posture, slouch, sit at a desk all day, or do a lot of traveling, you may want to consider checking with your physician or physical therapist about purchasing a lumbar roll.

Lumbar rolls are available through Orthopedic Physical Therapy Products in Minneapolis, Minnesota.

Do You Recommend a Chiropractor for a Back Injury?

Here we go again. That's just like asking me, if someone has a chronic headache, would I recommend that person see his or her family physician, a brain specialist, a neurologist, an oncologist, or an allergist? Generally speaking, your best bet is to see your family physician first, for both the chronic headache and the back injury.

In answer to the original question, I would recommend a chiropractor in some cases, and in others I would not. It depends on the type of back injury that we're talking about. If the condition is one in which your "back is out" or malaligned and requires manipulation to correct a displacement, certainly one might consider consulting a good chiropractor. What ultimately has to be kept in mind is that *chiropractic manipulation is not for every back problem.* Unfortunately, there are some chiropractors who feel that most back problems can be treated with spinal manipulation. If only it was that simple! A thorough examination needs to be done beforehand to determine whether a patient will benefit from manipulation.

Secondly, chiropractors do much more than merely "crack" backs. Their treatment goals are also the complete treatment of a patient. They are, however, not allowed to prescribe medication.

Thirdly, unfortunately many M.D.s and chiropractors do not have the best of working relationships. Many physicians do not recognize the work of chiropractors, and are therefore reticent to refer a patient to a chiropractor. The truth of the matter is that both should work together.

Last but not least, even though chiropractors and physicians have their own areas of expertise, many of these areas do overlap. Their goals are basically the same, with some emphasizing preventive care more than others. Obviously, if a CAT scan, prescription medication, laser treatment, or surgery are required, see an M.D. If a condition is borderline and could be treated by either a physician or a chiropractor, my recommendation is to see a physican first. Also keep in mind that there are many excellent physical therapists who have specialized in manual therapy. Whatever you do, keep in mind that chiropractors, just as physicians, have good and bad within their ranks. Seek out the best.

Do You Recommend Inversion (Hanging Upside Down)?

Yes I do, but not to everyone. I have worked with one of the gravity units for the last twelve years and have found it to be very helpful for many people suffering from back problems. However, there are also many back sufferers who have used it without success, or with very little success. Getting well really depends on the following factors:

1. What is the extent of the back injury?
2. Is the injury chronic or acute?
3. Is the pain centralized (localized) or is there peripheralization (pain radiating to the extremities)?
4. Type of treatment and frequency.
5. Individual's desire to get well.

Check with your physician before getting on any of these units.

What Does It Do? The primary purpose of a gravity unit is for spinal decompression or intervertebral separation. This is just a fancy way of saying that it stretches the back and separates the spinal vertebra. With your physicians approval, it might also be used for:

1. Herniated or degenerative discs
2. Sciatica or other neurological (nerve) inflammation
3. Muscle spasm
4. Pronounced lordosis (swayback)
5. Scoliosis (lateral curvature of the spine)
6. Relaxation
7. Increase cervical, thoracic, and lumbar flexibility

Who Should Not Use The Gravity Units? This is a very important question. Unfortunately, many of these gravity units are being used very indiscriminately without monitoring or supervision. Many people are put on these units who should not be on them. Health clubs and sporting good stores are two of the biggest offenders. Anyone with any of the following conditions is advised *not* to use the gravity units:

1. Cerebral vascular accident (stroke)
2. Congestive heart failure
3. Recent back surgery
4. Seizure disorders
5. Vertigo (dizziness)
6. Bone cancer
7. Hypertension (high blood pressure)
8. Angina pectoris (chest pain caused by insufficient blood supply to the heart).
9. Heart murmur
10. Meniere's disease (an ear condition characterized by progressive deafness, ringing in the ears, dizziness, and a sensation of fullness or pressure in the ears).
11. Thrombophlebitis (inflammation of a vein in conjunction with the formation of a blood clot or thrombus. The blood clot usually occurs in an extremity, most frequently a leg).
12. Hiatus hernia
13. Retinal detachment (an abnormal eye condition).
14. Glaucoma (disease of the eye characterized by an increase in pressure within the eye which results in atrophy of the optic nerve and blindness).
15. Pregnancy
16. Pulmonary disease
17. Obesity

How Long Should One Hang Upside Down? Assuming there are no medical restrictions, the length of time will vary from person to person. Initially, I would recommend hanging for about 1-2 minutes or as tolerated. After that, each person can gradually increase hanging time. I should also add that some people are unable to tolerate more than a few seconds during some of the initial attempts. Disorientation while hanging upside down is common.

CHAPTER 5 NOTES

[1] Knox, Richard A., "Low Back Pain is a Miserable Problem for Millions," *Los Angeles Times,* Part VII, April 5, 1981, p. 2.

[2] *Ibid.*

[3] McKenzie, Robin, *Treat Your Own Back* (Waikanae, New Zealand: Spinal Publications, 1980), p. 13.

[4] Grant, Arthur, *Back Care* (Bellvue, Washington: Medic Publishing Co., 1975), p. 10.

[5] Kraus, Hans, "Diagnosis and Management of Back Pain," *Weekly Anesthesiology Update,* Vol. II, Lesson 38, 1979.

[6] Micheli, L.J., Jackson, D.W., Stanish, W., "Symposium on Low Back Pain in Athletes," *American Journal of Sports Medicine,* VII: 361-9, 1979.

[7] McKenzie, Robin, *Treat Your Own Back* (Waikanae, New Zealand: Spinal Publications, 1980), pp. 11, 12, 14.

[8] *Ibid.*

[9] *Ibid.*

[10] Martin, Robert, *The Gravity Guiding System,* (Pasadena, California: Gravity Guidance, Inc., 1982). p. 42.

[11] Crouch, James E., *Functional Human Anatomy* (Philadelphia: Lea & Febiger, 1973), p. 126.

[12] Keim, Hugo A., "Low Back Pain," *CIBA Clinical Symposia,* Vol. XXV, No. 3: 14-16, 1973.

[13] *Taber's Cyclopedic Medical Dictionary* (F.A. Davis Co., 1977), p. S-22.

[14] McKenzie, Robin, *The Lumbar Spine, Mechanical Diagnosis and Therapy* (Waikanae, New Zealand: Spinal Publications, 1981), pp. 91-2.

[15] *Ibid.*

[16] *Ibid.*

[17] *Ibid.*

[18] *Ibid.*

[19] *Ibid.*

Chapter 6

DEFINITION

The only restrictions and limitations in life are those which we create for ourselves.

—David Luna

I don't want to be "smooth." How do I get "ripped?" How do I get "cut up?" These are questions I hear very often from men as well as women, and they all mean the same thing—definition. What is definition? Definition is the end result of a training and dietary program that enables you to visibly show muscle separation. Muscle separation is not something that is achieved overnight. It usually requires years of training and conditioning and fewer visits to Jack in the Box, McDonald's, and Haagen Daz Ice Cream Shoppes.

Many people feel that, if they become massive, they'll automatically obtain definition. The truth of the matter is that one can develop muscularity and still be smooth as silk. If the layer of fat is too thick, no matter how big the muscles are, you will not expose individual muscle fibers or muscle groups. Conversely, if you diet to try to obtain definition and do not exercise, you're not only going to lose fat, but also lean body mass (muscle). If you need to lose weight and want definition, do it through diet and exercise combined.

If you're still with me and you want to develop definition, here's what to do:

Lower Your Body Fat

Body fat is like a blanket. It can either be thick or thin, or somewhere in between. The thinner the blanket is, the more exposure to lean body mass underneath. The only advantages of having a high percentage of body fat are that you can float in water and be warm in winter.

The following are a few norms that will enable you to make a comparative analysis:

Body Fat Ratios

1. Most men average between 12 and 24 percent body fat. An ideal percentage of body fat for most men is less than 17 percent.
2. Most women average between 15 and 38 percent body fat. An ideal percentage would be 20 to 23 percent. It is not recommended that women drop below 17 percent. Dr. Karen Bradshaw, a researcher in obstetrics and gynecology at Tufts University Medical School in

Boston, suggests that in order to produce estrogen, a woman must maintain a level of body fat that is over 17 percent of her total weight. The young woman who is about to begin puberty needs at least 17 percent to develop breasts and to start a normal menstrual cycle.[1]

Range of Values of Relative Body Fat

Male distance runner	4-8%
Male gymnast	4-8%
Female distance runner	8-13%
Average college-aged male	13-16%
Average college-aged female	23-26%
Sedentary 40-year-old man	21-25%
Sedentary 40-year-old woman	30-36%

Maintain Ideal Body Weight

The formula we use for determining ideal body weight is described in Chapter 8 on page 87.

Exercise

Without exercise, definition is difficult to attain. Exercise accentuates and enhances every muscle fiber. The type of exercise recommended for definition is that which utilizes or integrates large muscle fiber recruitment over a sustained period of time. Large muscle fiber recruitment involves the use of muscles such as legs, chest, and back, which burn more calories and subsequently more body fat.

Exercise also increases lean body mass (muscle) and metabolism, both of which burn more calories and body fat.

Aerobic Activity

Body fat is burned through aerobic metabolism. Activities such as walking, running, aerobic classes, cycling, stair training (Stairmaster), swimming, and rope-jumping are very helpful in this respect. An additional benefit of aerobic activity is the obvious improvement in endurance.

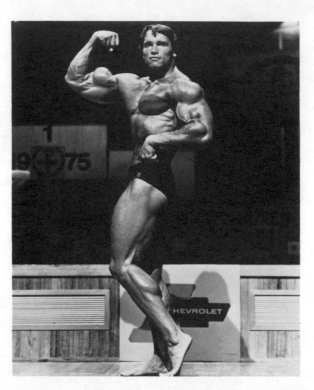

Figure 6-1. Arnold Schwarzenegger, All-time Greatest Bodybuilder, holder of 13 World Championship titles. *(Photo by Jimmy Caruso.)*

Circuit Weight Training

This is a practice that I highly recommend, because of the intense muscular demands. It is based on moving from one weight training station to another within a specified period of time. The rest phase between stations is generally 30 to 60 seconds. Circuit weight training is for those at an intermediate or advanced level.

Isolation

During training, it is important to isolate each body part and eliminate inertia (momentum) as much as possible. Muscle fiber recruitment through strictly executed movement is an absolute essential. Arnold Schwarzenegger points out, "Total muscle separation is the result of training each muscle so thoroughly that every plane, contour, and aspect is brought out and fully revealed once you have lowered your body fat sufficiently. To achieve this requires many different exercises for each muscle and a lot of

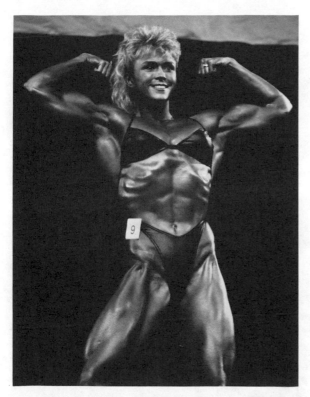

Figure 6-2. Tonya Knight, Miss International 1987 and Miss Olympia Contender. *(Photo by Art Zeller.)*

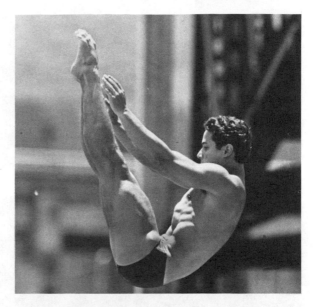

Figure 6-3. Greg Louganis, 1984 and 1988 Olympic Gold Medalist. *(Photo courtesy of Babbitt Productions, Malibu, CA.)*

sets and repetitions. The utmost muscle separation cannot be achieved without strictness of movement involving concentrated effort through the entire range of motion of the exercise, so that every engaged fiber is subjected to the maximum amount of stress. Any sloppiness of execution will defeat your purpose."[2]

Cross-training

Cross-training or the variety conditioning concept is based on integrating two or three different activities such as weight training, running, and/or aerobics classes into your workout program. The choices are optional. The purpose is threefold: (a) it permits you to work muscle groups from different angles and variations; (b) it keeps your program interesting and diversified; and (c) you're not stressing or traumatizing the same joints or muscle groups over and over again.

Implement a Low-Fat, High Complex-Carbohydrate Diet

Traditionally, most body builders have relied on a low carbohydrate, high-protein diet for definition. Essentially what this does is deplete glycogen reserves (stored energy) in the muscle and liver and utilizes fat and protein as sources of energy. Many diets are based on this concept. They have just been given different names. The disadvantages to these diets are that they are: (a) unbalanced; (b) high in fat; and (c) undesirable for long-term use, because they may be associated with degenerative diseases such as heart disease, strokes, and gall bladder problems. Therefore, place more emphasis on vegetables, fruits, grains, non-fat dairy products, and baked or broiled fish and poultry. Avoid foods that are fried and high in fat, cholesterol, and salt.

A WORD OF CAUTION

There are presently two practices that have come into vogue for obtaining definition, which I do not recommend. The first is based on the use of caffeine, a stimulant, to spare glycogen (stored

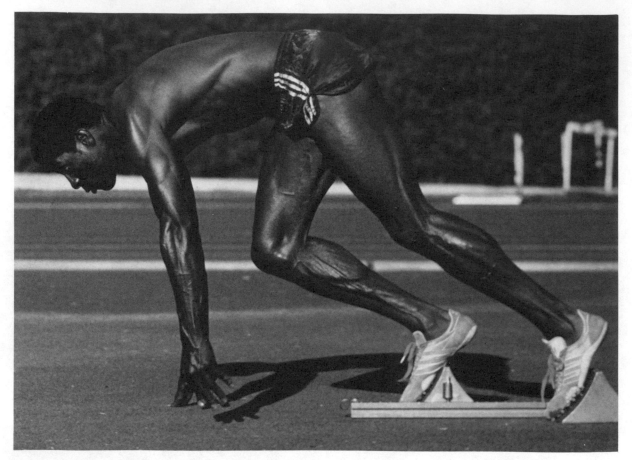

Figure 6-4. John Smith, 1972 Olympian World Record Holder, 440 yards (44:50) *(Photo by Mike Neveux.)*

energy), and increase free fatty acid utilization. This practice is based on decreasing body fat and increasing endurance. Current studies indicate that the efficacy of this practice is questionable at best. The second practice is "getting the water out" of the subcutaneous tissue to accentuate definition, resulting in a look that is less puffy and gives the muscles a tighter look. Any discipline that involves dehydration, or a conscious withholding of fluids or the use of diuretics, for competitive purposes or otherwise, does not meet with my seal of approval or of any competent fitness advisor.

One other practice I'd like to comment on: Fitness Professionals of America does not recommend the use of substances such as anabolic steroids or human growth hormones. The risks by far outweigh the benefits.

Definition is the ultimate goal in body building. It is the *creme de la creme*—the finishing touches on a piece of sculpture, though it is not something that one attains in a few weeks or months. In most cases, it takes years to develop. So be patient, train hard, and eat right, because the road ahead will be a long but worthy journey.

CHAPTER 6 NOTES

[1] "Estrogen and Your Health," *The Aerobics News,* Institute for Aerobics Research, Dallas, Texas, Vol II, No. 12, December 1987, p. 7.

[2] Schwarzenegger, Arnold, *Encyclopedia of Modern Body Building* (New York: Simon and Schuster, 1985), p. 197.

Part II

THE LUNA
DIET

Chapter 7

BEHAVIORAL MODIFICATION

Any dietary program without behavioral modification is a waste of time.

—David Luna

"Lose 30 pounds in thirty days on new crash diet! Clinically tested. Medically proven!"

"Eat all you want and still lose 5 pounds per day! No exercise, no hunger pains!"

How many times have you opened a newspaper or magazine to read headlines like these? How many times have you heen tempted to try one of these programs? Or better yet, how many times have you actually gone on one of these quick weight-loss programs with the hope that you would finally be able to control your weight? How many times have you been depressed or just plain fed up with going on one diet and off another? How many times have you been angry and upset at yourself for not being able to be in control, or disappointed because you're still having trouble keeping the weight off. How many times have you said to yourself, "I have to get my act together!"

The word "diet" is associated with many negative emotions—words like "depression," "frustration," "deprivation," "hopelessness," "regimentation," "anger," and "disappointment" come to mind. The first three letters of the word "diet" are certainly not very encouraging—D-I-E! The word diet, sometimes abbreviated to mean, "Did I Eat That?" has very negative connotations. One of the purposes of this book is to let you know that it doesn't have to be that way. It's always much better to light one candle than to curse the darkness. It is hoped that, by the time you finish reading this book, you'll be able to light a few candles.

The following information will center on showing you how the Luna Diet and behavioral modification can be applied in a sensible way without experiencing any of the negative feelings and emotions associated with most dietary programs. It will give you a better insight and understanding of your eating behaviors and also show you techniques on how to change some of those undesirable behaviors. Most of us only have a vague awareness of what we eat and how we eat, thus the emergence of behavioral modification.

What is behavioral modification? It is the systematic substitution of one set of behaviors for another by selectively rewarding the desired behaviors. However, *before you can change behaviors, you must change attitude.*

If the right attitude is not present, then it doesn't matter what kind of program you're on. Your chances of succeeding are not in your favor. Any program that does not integrate behavioral modification and attitude changes is a waste of time. It becomes vitally important for you to understand what you're doing and why. Otherwise, your program becomes a redundant rehearsal of errors.

Behavioral modification is not only interested

in what you have consumed, but also how much, when, where, the physical position, how you felt, the degree of hunger, and associated activity. All of this information is then recorded into a food journal to make you aware of how much you're eating, and also to look for specific patterns that might be causing problems. Make special notes of problem times, problem situations, and worst temptations, so you can avoid them. Foods should be noted in the journal or diary shortly after being consumed, rather than waiting until the end of the day to write in everything. Too much may be omitted or forgotten between morning and evening.

If you're working in conjunction with a weight-reduction specialist, dietitian, or nutritional consultant, the food journal can be used for a more in-depth analysis and evaluation of eating habits. All the clients I have on weight-reduction programs keep daily food journals. I would recommend you do the same. Make reproductions of the food journal in Table VII-1

so you can start noting your daily food consumption.

RECOMMENDATIONS FOR BEHAVIORAL WEIGHT-CONTROL PROGRAM

Even though each person should be considered on an individual basis, the following are general recommendations for behavioral modification as they relate to the Luna Diet:

Behavioral Modification at Home

1. Plan your meals in advance. I once had a client who would take up to two hours to decide what she was going to eat. Too much time wasted on indecision. Decide in advance.
2. Sit down and eat slowly.

THE LUNA DIET FOOD JOURNAL

Name _____ Weight beginning of week_____

Date _____ Weight end of week_____

Activities While Eating (AWE)
0-None   3-Reading
1-Watching TV 4-Driving
2-Working   5-Talking on
                          Telephone

Hunger Level On A Ratio From 1-4
1-No Hunger
2-Some Hunger
3-Normal Hunger
4-Very Hungry

Body Position (BP)
1-Sitting
2-Standing
3-Walking
4-Lying Down

Eating With Whom
A-Alone   F-Family
BA-Business   FD-Friend
            Associate R-Relative
C-Children   S-Spouse

Eating Location
A-Automobile   K-Kitchen
B-Bedroom   LR-Living Room
C-Cafeteria   R-Restaurant
D-Desk   W-Work
DR-Dining Room

Feelings Before Eating
A-Angry   I-Indifferent
B-Bored   N-Neutral
D-Depressed   R-Rushed
F-Fat   S-Sad
FD-Frustrated T-Tension
G-Great   TN-Thin
H-Happy   TD-Tired

*PA-Physical Activity For The Day

Feelings After Eating
F-Full   S-Satisfied
G-Guilty   SK-Sick
H-Hungry   SD-Stuffed
O-OK   T-Terrible

Date	Meal	Hunger Level	List All Foods Consumed	Total Liquids Consumed	BP	AWE	Time Spent Eating	Eating Location	Eating With Whom	Feelings Before Eating	Feelings After Eating	PA*
	Breakfast											
	Lunch											
	Dinner											
	Snack											
	Breakfast											
	Lunch											
	Dinner											
	Snack											

3. Stay away from the kitchen or any problem areas.

4. Avoid activities, such as watching TV or reading, while eating. There's a tendency to become engrossed with the activity and lose awareness of how much you're consuming.

5. Avoid eating finger foods. Try to eat most of your meals with a knife and fork. If you're going to eat a sandwich, eat it with a knife and fork.

6. Cut food as it is needed.

7. Put your knife and fork down while the food is in your mouth.

8. Allow yourself a few interruptions during each meal.

9. Keep tempting foods out of sight. ("Out of sight, out of mind.")

10. If you don't want tempting foods around, *don't buy tempting foods.* If it's your splurge for the week, then either buy a small portion or a small amount of the desired food. (For example, one-fourth of a small pie instead of a whole pie, or a pint of ice cream instead of a half gallon.) Don't make it any more difficult on yourself than you have to.

11. Don't clean your plate if you're not hungry.

12. Remove your plate, whether or not there's anything left on it, as soon as you have finished eating. Even though you may be full, there's always a tendency to continue nibbling on leftover food or to indulge in second helpings.

13. Never eat standing up. Sit down and use utensils. Eating while standing may make your meal seem like a snack.

14. Have low-calorie foods such as fresh vegetables, fresh fruit, and unsalted crackers available (preferably in the front of the refrigerator).

15. Use smaller plates and glasses, along with smaller servings.

16. Don't eat every meal as though there's no tomorrow.

17. Politely refuse offers for extra servings if you've consumed enough food to meet your needs.

18. Involve other people: family, friends, and colleagues, and ask for their cooperation.

Leftovers

There are several things you can do to reduce the risk of overeating because of leftovers. Consider some of these suggestions:

1. No matter how much food is leftover, if you're not hungry, put whatever food that is leftover in the refrigerator, and eat it later when you are hungry. It doesn't matter how small the amount is, save it or throw it out. On many occasions, I have put small amounts of food into the refrigerator when I no longer wanted any more rather than "packing it in." It takes time, training, patience, and awareness to learn this behavior.

2. Some experts recommend pouring salt, pepper, or hot-sauce over unwanted leftovers. I don't feel this is necessary, but if it helps you, use it.

3. Remove serving dishes from the table as soon as you have finished eating.

Behavioral Modification at Work

The work environment presents a wide variety of opportunities for unplanned eating. Here are some examples that should prove to be helpful.

1. Don't eat while you're working. You may become so involved mentally and emotionally with your work that you may lose track of how much you're eating.

2. Don't keep tempting foods (chocolates, cookies, candy, etc.) in your desk drawers.

3. Pre-package food "emergency kits" for times when you are upset, depressed, lonely, angry, or likely to get out of control.[1]

4. Don't buy food from vending machines and fast-food restaurants.

5. If you're going out to lunch with your co-workers, plan your order; order first; order *a la carte;* ask for water; and systematically undereat.

6. *Taxi and truck drivers:* don't eat and drive

at the same time. *Culinary workers and cooks:* don't nibble on your specials during your shift. *Secretaries:* the "goodies" that you have stashed away in your desk drawer may be walking and talking tomorrow. *Doctors:* if you want to advise your patients more effectively about their diets, set a good example. *Housewives:* don't eat the junk food because the children insist on having it around the house. *Nurses:* Don't eat the "goodies" because the patient refused them.

Behavioral Modification in Restaurants

Eating out is fun, and that aspect shouldn't have to change just because you're on a diet. Author Julie Waltz uses the motto, *"Get the best of what there is, not all of what there is,"* as the approach to use when eating out. Here are some things you can do when you are in a restaurant.

1. Plan your order ahead of time.
2. Avoid starving yourself all day in anticipation of the dinner meal. Eat a little snack before you leave (if you feel it's necessary) so you won't arrive hungry.
3. Order first, so you won't be swayed by what anyone else orders.
4. Order vegetables or a small salad and water before you even read the menu.
5. Order *a la carte* to get exactly what you want.
6. Order in accordance with your level of hunger.
7. Share your food with others, particularly high-calorie foods.
8. Always ask for your salad dressing on the side. Use low-calorie dressings like herb, lemon or plain vinegar.
9. If you only want one pat of butter, request it. If you don't want jam on the table, ask the waiter or waitress to remove it. Better yet, pass on both.
10. Slow down. Even though everyone all around you may be rushing or gulping down their food, repeat, "I am in control," and eat in slow motion.
11. As soon as you've finished eating, have the waiter remove any leftover food. Another option is to have the food put in a "dieter's bag."
12. Avoid restaurants that offer all you can eat for a set price. Everyone always wants to get their money's worth, so they inevitably end up eating more than they normally eat.
13. Be selective about the restaurants you patronize. Go to restaurants where you know you'll get the type of food you want and make sure it is well prepared. Avoid fast-food restaurants. They may be convenient and inexpensive, but much of the food is too high in fat and calories. I would suggest that you *not* patronize the following restaurants:

> The Greasy Spoon
> Ptomaine Harry's
> The Scarf and Barf
> Trash at the Top
> Botulism Bob's
> Pepe Bismol's
> The Dysentery Inn
> Turista Delight Cafe
> Fred's Fatburger
> Hy Cholesterol's Delicatessen
> Le Garbawge Cafe
> Run's Fast Foods
> Saltine Sally's
> Mylanta Inn
> Yuckies Pizza Parlor
> The Sleeze Bucket Cafe

Business Luncheons

One of the biggest problems faced by all of us in the business world are business luncheons, also known as the "three-martini lunch." How do we take out clients to "wine and dine" them and not overindulge ourselves? Well, I have several suggestions you could keep in mind when you are faced with this dilemma:

1. Order your cocktail after your client orders his. Then ask for a mineral water back-up. When your drinks arrive, have a toast, take a sip, then "nurse" the sparkling

water for the remainder of the luncheon. Your cocktail, in essence, becomes more of a theatrical prop. If your client notices that you're not "keeping up" with him, simply say, "I've had enough." In a professional atmosphere, this should suffice. Then it's business as usual.

2. The main thing to keep in mind here is that no one likes to eat and drink alone. Therefore, order anything you like that's consistent with your usual eating patterns. But remember—you do not have to eat everything that is ordered. Shift the focus of attention to business. That is, after all, why you're there.

Shopping

Here are some general rules you might keep in mind when you go shopping.

1. Don't shop when you're hungry. You may buy things you'll regret later.
2. Shop from a specific list.
3. Read labels.
4. As you roll the shopping cart down the aisles, remind yourself of your projected weight goal and that you want quality food for "fuel."
5. If you take your children shopping with you, don't let them influence you into buying foods that are going to be difficult for you to deal with. Good nutrition starts in the home and at an early age.
6. If you buy a "treat food" such as cookies or ice cream (hopefully not too often), purchase the smallest package or container available.
7. Don't munch on the groceries on the way home.

Emergency Food Kits

A good idea when you're watching your diet is to keep healthy, low-calorie foods handy, in case you run into any emergency situations. Here are some examples:

1. *Vegetable/cracker kit:* fill a plastic bag with carrot sticks, cherry tomatoes, small cucumbers, cauliflower, or broccoli florets with unsalted whole-wheat crackers on the side.
2. *Tomato sandwich kit:* Take one slice of whole wheat, rye, or pumpernickel bread and cut it in half. Add one leaf of romaine lettuce and two slices of tomato. What, no meat? No meat.
3. *Fresh fruit kit:* Pack a couple of pieces of fruit.
4. *Rice cake and grape kit:* pack a few rice cakes (dried brown rice) and some fresh grapes. Combine the two for a great picker-upper.
5. *Non-fat yogurt and fresh strawberry kit:* take a small container of plain, non-fat yogurt and mix with fresh strawberries or sliced banana.
6. *The raisin kit:* pack one small box of raisins.
7. *Trail mix kit:* since nuts are high in calories, use this kit sparingly. Combine a few unsalted, unprocessed peanuts, almonds, or sunflower seeds with some raisins.

Remember, eating anything to excess will cause you to gain weight, so use these kits sensibly. You may also want to consider carrying a couple of herbal tea bags—to replace the coffee in your diet.

HINTS FOR GOOD HEALTH AND WEIGHT LOSS

Here are some additional guidelines to use in conjunction with the Luna Diet:

1. *Develop Systematic Undereating:* This is an eating concept based on eating approximately 5% - 10% less of what you might normally eat. When you get up from a meal, you don't want to be hungry, yet you don't want to be stuffed.

2. *Food is Fuel:* So just eat when you're hungry; don't eat at 12:00 simply because it's lunchtime or 6:00 because it's dinnertime if you're not hungry.

3. *Take Charge:* The way you eat is a reflection of how much control you really have in your life. Be in command, and fulfill your destiny. You can do anything you want once you've made the commitment.

4. *Be Aware:* Even though you're not counting calories on the Luna Diet, be aware of the caloric and fat content of foods.

5. *Drink Water:* When you can, replace soft drinks, coffee, tea, and especially alcohol with water; it has no calories, no fat, no cholesterol, and it's great for your skin.

6. *Don't Starve Yourself:* It's a self-defeating way to try to lose weight. Dorothy Dusek, Ph.D, and author of the book, *Thin and Fit: Your Personal Lifestyle,* explains that, "As you decrease your energy input below an obligatory level, your body's metabolic rate *decreases,* so it becomes harder to utilize the foods you do allow yourself. This is the basic conservation of energy law designed by nature for our survival."

   Dr. Dusek also adds that, "If when trying to lose weight, you decrease your intake to, say, fewer than 1000 calories per day, that severe denial of food will cause your body to shut down because it wants to survive. The body seems to know it isn't being fed much, so it reduces the amount of energy that it would normally produce. Also, when you starve yourself, you lose muscle mass, so there is less lean tissue to metabolize the fat you're trying to get rid of."

   Starvation, according to Dr. Dusek, (a) decreases metabolic rate, (b) seriously limits the intake of vital nutrients, especially protein, vitamins, and minerals, all of which can be vital to weight-loss, and (c) promotes self-defeat, which makes you rather cranky about life in general.

7. *Enjoy Your Meal:* But also keep in mind that it only takes twenty minutes for your stomach to send your brain the message that it's full, so take your time.

8. *Don't Clean Your Plate:* If you're not hungry, don't eat. Most of us have been psychologically conditioned since childhood to eat everything on our plates. We were constantly reminded by our parents that people were starving throughout the world and we'd be wasting food if we didn't "clean our plates." Guilt (and in some cases obesity) was often the result of this early message. Some simple solutions to this syndrome are: (a) serve smaller portions; (b) if you're not hungry, put leftovers in the refrigerator to eat later; (c) if you're eating out, stop when you are full. I realize this is easier said than done; however, it can be done by understanding behavorial shaping, making a strong commitment, and again by systematic undereating.

9. *Commit and Have Confidence in Yourself:* Don't just try, go for it. Trying is a tentative thing. It's too borderline. It's too lukewarm. Even though I never fault anyone for trying, the commitment has just got to be more affirmative to work. For example, say, "I'm going to lose the weight," instead of "I'm going to try to lose the weight." Olympic sprinter Carl Lewis once said, "If you don't have confidence, you'll always find a way not to win."

10. *Place Your Scale in Front of or Beside Your Refrigerator:* This will help keep tabs on your progress. One word of caution: beware of developing a fixation with the scale. If you find yourself weighing in several times during the day, such as after a meal, before a meal, or after you've gone to the bathroom, then you've carried the practice to an extreme. Neurotic scale fixations are not a part of this program. Weigh in once a week, and that's it. Any more than that, no matter how great the temptation, is to be avoided. Otherwise, the scale may start playing games with your mind. If you find you've

developed a fixation with the scale, limit your "weigh-ins" to once every two weeks. The remainder of the time, you will have to depend on your clothes and the self-evaluation you do in front of the mirror in your "birthday suit" to determine your progress.

Also be aware of fluctuations in your weight that may exist as a result of fluid retention and not necessarily overconsumption. *Women:* Be particularly aware of this during your menstrual cycle, so you won't be devastated if your weight increases a few pounds in spite of the systematic undereating and increased physical activity. There's no need for concern over an occasional isolated incident, but there is concern for what the graph might show over an extended period of time. Is the weight progressively decreasing, increasing, or on a holding pattern?

Another reason for weighing in once a week is because you're not counting calories or carbohydrates. The scale, your clothes, a bodyfat evaluation, and a visual examination of yourself in your "birthday suit" are valid criteria that will enable you to determine whether or not the program is working.

One final point about weighing in: try to weigh in around the same time of the day whenever possible.

11. *Keep a Journal:* Of everything you've eaten. This enables you to become aware of how much you're eating, as well as what you're eating. (See Table VII-1.)
12. *Use Visualization:* Visualize your goals, and set the stage for success. If you think success, you create a climate in which success is probable. If you think failure, you set the stage for it.
13. *Set Goals:* Write all your intermediate and long-range goals, then sign and date the list.
14. *Take One Day and One Meal at a Time:* No one is ever good 100% of the time.

15. *Eat to Please Yourself, Not Others:* Just about everyone, at one time or another, has eaten something they didn't want merely to please someone else. Don't get caught in that trap. Stay with your game plan.
16. *Take a Photograph:* Have someone take a photograph of you in a swimsuit and place it in front of your bedroom mirror or on the refrigerator door. Photographs don't lie. Another option is to put up a photograph of someone you'd like to look like with a similar body type or build.
17. *Chew Gum:* If you need something to keep your mouth busy, chew sugarless gum.
18. *Avoid Rationalizations and Bad Environmental Planning:* An example of this is someone who says, "If I eat this box of cookies today, I won't have them around to tempt me tomorrow."
19. *Use Positive Reinforcement:* Compliment yourself for a job well-done, rather than depending on others to compliment you (external positive reinforcement). The problem with external positive reinforcement is that you may come to depend on compliments from others and eventually expect it. Learn to depend on yourself. Also, positive reinforcement is more effective in establishing a behavior than negative reinforcement has in getting rid of it. Positive reinforcement is four times more effective.
20. *Use Your Own Decision-making Process:* When you sit down to have a meal, at some point you're going to have to make a conscious decision about when to stop. This process is an important one, for it will dictate whether you succeed, remain on a holding pattern, or fail.
21. *Don't Be Influenced Negatively by the Media:* Beware of T.V. commercials about food that might catch you at a weak moment. The power of suggestion can be very strong, and that's why I suggest you have some low-calorie snacks readily available. Advertisers are no dummies

when it comes to your tummy.

22. *Individualize and Deal with Your Own Circumstances:* There's no such thing as normal eating habits; they're different for everyone; dieting is, has been, and always will be individualized.

CHAPTER 7 NOTES

[1] Julie Waltz, *Food Habit Management,* Northwest Learning Associates, Inc., Seattle, Washington, 1978, pp. 267-269.

Chapter 8

THE LUNA DIET
A LONG-RANGE PROGRAM
FOR BETTER NUTRITION

Success is that place in the road where preparation and opportunity meet. However, very few people recognize it, because it very often comes disguised as hard work.

We live in a land of overabundance, and, in the area of health, "more" often means "less." Dr. William Glasser, author of *Positive Addiction,* writes:

> The simple statement we sometimes say out loud, but more often say to ourselves: "The heck with it," means we are settling for less, because we don't have it in us now to struggle for more. We settle for less with our marriages, our children, our employers, and our neighbors than we know we should. We drink, we smoke, we eat too much and too many of the wrong kinds of foods, because it's easier than disciplining ourselves to say no. I am not recommending that we should be more rigid or contentious, for that too is weakness. It takes strength, however, to be warm, firm, humorous, and caring and still do what we know we ought to do. Our lives would be much better if we never said "The heck with it."[1]

Getting people to change their eating behaviors is a difficult task. We're basically creatures of habit, and therefore look for the easy way out. It's much easier to say, "The heck with it." But we may not be able to go on saying that

indefinitely, for everything in life catches up with us eventually, especially the "skeletons" in our closets.

As president of Fitness Professionals of America, I frequently hear some of the following comments:

"I'm having trouble getting my act together."
"I'm tired of having problems with my weight. I don't want to have to struggle with it the rest of my life."
"What difference does it make? I'm too old to exercise."
"I don't feel good about myself."
"I finally took a good, hard look at myself, after abusing and neglecting myself for a long time, and I didn't like what I saw."
"If I only knew then what I know now."

Nearly everyone has experienced one or more of these feelings at some time or other. However, the bottom line is that life does not have to be that way. It doesn't have to be a series of regrets and disappointments. When things go wrong, you don't have to go with them. You can be in control of your life, if that's what you decide.

Infectious agents are always present in our environment. However, they are under control if we maintain our natural health and a strong immune response (resistance to disease). This, unfortunately, is where many of us fail, and when we do, the "bugs" are ready to step in and do damage as soon as the resistance is lowered. By practicing preventive medicine and becoming "positively addicted" to exercise and good nutrition, you can gradually begin to lower some of the risk factors for disease while simultaneously increasing your level of resistance. This might be timely advice considering the current health epidemic with AIDS, which is spreading throughout the world. At the present time, one person per minute is contracting this fatal disease worldwide. Even if there is no cure for AIDS, it would be in all our best interests to maintain a high level of resistance.

Dr. Kenneth Cooper, medical director of the Aerobics Institute in Dallas, Texas, recently pointed out that he had not missed work due to illness in over 27 years. Most of us would be doing well if we only missed one or two days a year due to illness. Dr. Cooper attributes his excellent health and apparent protection from infectious disease to several factors evolving around lifestyle, one of which is his regular aerobics program. Good health and a strong immune system do not happen by accident. A good diet and a moderate exercise program can help you to build and strengthen your level of resistance.

The Luna Diet presented here is a broad, preventive nutritional plan, designed as a guideline for establishing a lifelong pattern of eating, as well as the understanding of eating behaviors. Do not think of this diet in terms of what you will have to give up, but rather what you will gain from it. Whether your dietary modifications are on a large or small scale will depend on your present patterns. Basically, all you will be doing is eliminating those foods that either don't have any nutritional value or very little nutritional value and replacing these items with foods that are nutritious. The only *exception* to eating the foods recommended in the Luna Diet is if you are allergic or hypersensitive to a specific food or food group.

The foods listed in Table VIII-1 are most commonly implicated in causing hypersensitive reactions.

Table VIII-1
FOODS WHICH MAY CAUSE HYPERSENSITIVE REACTIONS

Eggs	Shellfish
Milk	Mollusks
Wheat	Beans
Peanuts	Yeast
Soybeans	Corn

If you discover that you might have an allergic reaction to any of these or other foods, you might be better off avoiding them. One of the problems with this, however, is that many times you may suspect a specific food but not really know for certain. If you suspect you may have either allergic reactions or digestive problems, consult a competent physician, board certified in allergy and immunology, before making any changes in your diet. Keep in mind that true food allergies are rare.

The Luna Diet will also help you to reduce some of the risk factors associated with degenerative disorders such as heart disease, diabetes, hypertension (high blood pressure), cerebral vascular disease (strokes), and certain forms of cancer.

The Luna Diet, with its emphasis on complex carbohydrates, can be used for weight loss. Complex carbohydrates are foods such as fruits, vegetables, whole grains, and legumes eaten as grown. They should not be confused with simple carbohydrates such as white sugar, brown sugar, honey, and molasses. There is no counting of calories involved, but there is an awareness of calories. *The weight loss occurs through the concept of Systematic Undereating, an awareness of actual hunger level, keeping a food journal, behavioral modification, and the Ultimate Fitness exercise program.*

The Luna Diet is also instrumental in preventing the proverbial "yo-yo syndrome." Most of the people whom I've counseled over the years have gone from one dietary program to another without success. You name it, they've tried it. Many go through an entire lifetime seeking the "ideal diet," even though there is no such thing—the Luna Diet included.

So what happens? You optimistically launch yourself into some popular diet. You feel very self-righteous for a few weeks, as you see your weight start to drop. Then, after you've lost as much weight as you need to prove to yourself that you can do it, you let the diet fall by the wayside, and you go back to your old eating habits. Inevitably, you put the pounds right back on again in less time than it took to lose them. What is happening ultimately, is that you're merely dealing with symptoms and not solutions. You haven't corrected the eating behaviors. It's like a coronary bypass. If you don't make the necessary changes in your diet following bypass or laser surgery, chances are it will be just a matter of time before the blood vessels are blocked again.

We know that 90 percent of the people who lose weight put it back on within a year. It doesn't have to be that way. But unfortunately, it doesn't matter which diet is followed; the pattern remains the same. How long can you eat only cottage cheese, lettuce, and alfalfa sprouts? How long are you going to keep track of the number of carbohydrates you consume per day? How long are you going to exist on appetite suppressants and water pills? How long are you going to remain on this physical and emotional roller coaster? The list of diets and weight-reduction aids goes on and on and will continue to do so until you understand the following: (1) *etiology*— the cause or causes; (2) *eating behaviors*— understanding and changing them; (3) *the food is fuel concept*—it can either be life-enhancing or life-diminishing; (4) *attitude*—it may have to change, particularly if your weight is becoming more difficult to control.

Losing the weight is not what's difficult. The hard part is keeping the weight off. The Luna Diet is designed with just this in mind. It's set up to help you prevent the "yo-yo syndrome" and to help you establish a lifelong dietary pattern based on *daily systematic undereating with a recommended weight loss of approximately 1 to 2 pounds per week*. Systematic Undereating is an eating concept based on eating approximately 5 to 10 percent less than what you normally eat. You don't get up from the table hungry, yet you're not full. Before you eat, ask yourself, "Am I hungry?" If you're not, then don't eat. If you're just a little hungry, have a small meal or snack. If you're very hungry, systematically undereat in accordance with your hunger level. It will take time, practice, and constant reinforcement before you develop this inner awareness of your actual hunger level. Otherwise, you may find yourself giving in to the whimsical dictates of: (a) the "robot" (the part of our subconscious that responds immediately and automatically to stimuli or directions we give it), (b) emotional eating, (c) the "binge" episode.

The Luna Diet uses the following formula for determining an ideal body weight for you:

1. For women, the first 5 feet are equivalent to the first 100 pounds, and every additional inch is equal to 5 pounds. Let's take a woman who is 64 inches in height (5′ 4″) as an example:

$$
\begin{array}{r}
\text{WOMEN } (e.g.\ 64'') \\
5' = 100 \text{ lbs.} \\
1'' = 5 \text{ lbs.} \\
\underline{\times\ 4 \text{ inches}} \\
= 20 \text{ lbs.}
\end{array}
$$

So, 100 + 20 = 120 lbs.

This would be the calculated ideal body weight, plus or minus 10 percent depending on body and size of frame.

2. For men, the first 5 feet are equivalent to 106 pounds, and every additional inch is equal to 6 pounds. Let's use for our example a man who is 71 inches in height (5′ 11″):

	Portion (oz.)	Total Fat (gms)	Protein (gms)	Calories	Iron (mg)
Table VIII-2 RED MEAT, FISH, AND POULTRY CHART*					
BEEF					
Sirloin	3.5	34.7	22.2	408	2.9
Steak	4.0	13.8	31.9	260	4.8
Chuck	3.5	9.5	30.0	214	3.8
Round	3.0	8.2	30.5	205	4.6
PORK					
Ham	3.5	11.0	18.0	175	0.9
Chop	3.5	25.6	29.4	357	4.4
CHICKEN					
Roasted with skin	3.5	10.9	29.0	222	1.1
Light, no skin	3.5	4.5	30.9	173	1.1
Dark, no skin	3.5	9.7	27.4	205	1.3
TURKEY					
Roasted with skin	3.5	8.3	28.6	197	1.4
Light no skin	3.5	3.2	29.9	157	1.3
Dark, no skin	3.5	7.2	28.6	187	2.3
TUNA					
In oil	3.25	11.0	23.5	193	0.9
In water	3.25	0.8	23.6	109	0.9
Cod (Broiled)	3.5	0.5	26.1	112	0.9
Salmon (Broiled)	3.5	7.4	27.0	182	1.2

Chart prepared by Ursula Weatherton, M.S., R.D., using Bowes & Church, Food Values of Portions Commonly Used, 14th ed. (Pennington & Church), 1985.

MEN (*e.g.* 71″)
5′ = 106 lbs.
1″ = 6 lbs.
× 11 inches
─────────
= 66 lbs.

So, 106 + 66 = 172 lbs.

This would be the calculated ideal body weight, plus or minus 10 percent depending on body and size of frame.

If your weight falls within these ranges, it is advised that you concentrate your efforts on maintaining the recommended body weight. Otherwise, if you are underweight or overweight, make the necessary adjustments gradually and accordingly.

Even if your goal is not to lose weight, but simply to maintain and stay fit, the Luna Diet will provide the basis for sound nutrition that can be maintained for a lifetime. The Luna Diet also makes every effort to provide you with the best and latest dietary information available. It also includes a list of foods that are recommended, a discussion of those food items to avoid, food additives, health hints, and easy-to-make recipes.

The following suggestion is optional: allow yourself *one* splurge per week. The splurge, as explained before, should be both *planned* and *controlled.* You decide what the splurge will be. This occasional reprieve will serve to eliminate any feelings of deprivation or depression that often accompany any major change in eating habits. It's a form of "ventilation" that enables you to diffuse, often avoiding, a major binge. After a while, you may find, to your surprise, that the junk foods you once relished are no longer as desirable as they were.

Work into these healthful eating habits gradually. Evolve into the new eating behaviors comfortably in order to adapt them to your own individual needs. Don't try to make too many changes at once. Your goal is to make lifelong changes in your eating habits to maintain optimum health and wellness.

RECOMMENDED FOODS

The following foods or food groups are recommended with the reservations indicated. Taken together, they form the basis for the Luna Diet plan. They are: (1) non-fat dairy products; (2) chicken, turkey, and fish in limited amounts; (3) vegetables and fruits; (4) whole grains, natural cereals, and brown breads, especially those high in fiber; (5) some selected nuts, seeds, and legumes.

Dairy Products

1. All dairy products should be non-fat. With regards to milk, infants under one year should be given regular milk or breast-fed. The reason skim milk or non-fat milk is considered all right for children (one year and over) but not infants, is that children are assumed to be eating a mixed diet and thus obtaining essential fatty acids such as linoleic acid from other sources. Non-fat milk does not contain linoleic acid. It is removed when the fat is taken out.

2. Skim cheese (in limited quantities).
3. Non-fat plain yogurt (not fruit flavored).
4. No egg yolks; all the egg whites desired; hard- or soft-boil eggs; don't eat eggs raw.

Fish and Poultry

Fish: Limit fish consumption to three times per week. Deemphasize shellfish. Besides being high in cholesterol, they're also scavengers.

Chicken and Turkey: Limit poultry to three times per week and don't fry it! Remove the skin and either bake or broil. Preferably consume white meat only (dark meat is higher in fat and calories).

Table VIII-2 will give you a good indication of why fish and chicken (or turkey) is preferred over red meat. Generally there are two reasons for this: there is less saturated fat, and there are fewer calories. Take a look for yourself at the comparisons the table gives.

Vegetables and Legumes

Vegetables and legumes are an excellent source of vitamins and minerals. So, eat a wide variety. Table VIII-3 provides examples of some of the best to include in your diet.

If you have a family history or a tendency to develop kidney stones, the following vegetables are high in oxalic acid and should either be avoided or eaten in limited quantities. They are: beet greens, rhubarb, spinach, and swiss chard.

Fruits

Fruits such as avacados and coconuts should generally be avoided. If you don't need to lose weight, you may eat as much fresh fruit as you like on the Luna Diet. Otherwise, practice the concept of Systematic Undereating.

Breads, Grains, and Cereal Products

Breads should either be dark or brown. Occasionally including bread such as sourdough French bread is okay. Natural grain cereals such as rolled oats and cracked wheat, which may be

Table VIII-3

VEGETABLES AND LEGUMES

You may select a variety of vegetables from the list below:

Alfalfa sprouts	Celery	Onions (careful— gasy)
Asparagus	Collard greens	Peas
Beans (careful—gasy)	Corn	Potatoes (not fried; include
	Cucumbers	skin; no gravy or sour cream)
Bean sprouts	Eggplant	Pumpkin
Broccoli (careful—gasy)	Green peppers	Radishes
Brussels sprouts (careful—gasy)	Jicama	Squash
Cabbage (careful—gasy)	Lettuce	Tomatoes
Carrots	Mushrooms	Turnip Greens
Cauliflower	Okra	Yams

Remember, never fry your vegetables; no sauces or butter; simply steam or eat fresh.

purchased in health food stores and most supermarkets, are recommended. The following commercial cereals are also recommended:

Quick Quaker Oats
Post Grapenuts
Kellogg's Nutri-Grain Corn
Kellogg's Nutri-Grain Wheat
Kellogg's Nutri-Grain Nuggets
Shredded Wheat
and a few of the cooked cereals

Most of the other commercially packaged breakfast cereals probably have more nutritional value in the box than the contents. Make it a habit to read labels. If the cereal product contains white or brown sugar, honey, or molasses, leave it on the shelf. Also, since cold cereals should be a low fat item, try to select those that contain no more than 10% of their calories from fat.

Fiber: The Roto Rooter that Doesn't Handle You Rough

Dietary fiber is that part of plant food that passes through the small intestine without being completely broken down by intestinal secretions and on into the large intestine virtually unchanged.

One of the functions of fiber is to stimulate peristalsis, the progressive "wormlike" movement of food in the intestinal tract. Fiber increases stool frequency and decreases transit time.

A high-fiber diet is one containing approximately 13 grams or more of crude fiber, while a restricted-fiber diet is one containing only 3 to 5 grams.[2] The daily adult requirement for fiber is aproximately 6 grams per day.[3] Diets low in fiber have been associated with an increased risk of heart disease, cancer of the colon, gallstones, diabetes, hiatus hernias, hemorrhoids, appendicitis, and diverticulitis.[4]

What Do You Recommend for Constipation?

The average person in the U.S. has a bowel movement about once every two days, whereas in Africa, for example, the Bantus and the Masai have two or three bowel movements in one day. The difference, according to many authorities, may lie in the consumption of more dietary fiber and the underconsumption of refined foods in these cultures, along with higher levels of activity.

Chronic constipation is generally due to lack of dietary fiber and exercise. One of the best sources of fiber is bran. Bran is inexpensive and can be purchased in any health food store. I do not recommend the commercial 100 percent bran cereals, because they usually contain refined sugar. Instead, take a tablespoon of wheat or oat bran and sprinkle it into a salad, a bowl of cereal, or into an energy drink made in a blender.

Additional causes of chronic constipation are: (a) insufficient water,[5] (b) worry and tension, (c) too many over-refined foods,[6] (d) high levels of fat and cholesterol,[7] and (e) postponement of bowel movements, which, incidently, is one of the principal causes of hemorrhoids.

Are you a Floater or a Sinker?

Dr. Denis P. Burkitt, a leading researcher of dietary fiber, has indicated that one manner of determining whether or not you're getting enough dietary fiber is by examining your stool. If the stool floats in water, then you're probably consuming enough fiber. However, if it doesn't, chances are that you're not, and are advised to increase dietary fiber intake.

Look at Table VIII-4 to get an idea of the levels of dietary fiber contained in everyday foods.

Is Dietary Fiber Beneficial for the Diabetic?

According to a recent article by Patricia Anastasio, R.D., in Environmental Nutrition, "Studies with diabetics have shown fiber to be helpful in minimizing the after eating rise in blood sugar and decreasing the demand on available insulin. Digestion and absorption take place over a longer period of time when fiber is present. The effects of fiber also appears to improve receptor sensitivity to insulin. High fiber diabetic diets are associated with less sugar in the urine, lower fasting blood sugar, and lower insulin requirements."[8]

Nuts and Seeds

Because of the high fat content, eat nuts and seeds sparingly. Preferably buy those that are unprocessed or unsalted.

Table VIII-4 FIBER LEVELS IN FOOD	
Sources of Fiber	*% Crude Fiber*
Bran	9.0
Dry Beans, Lentils	4.0
Nuts	2.0
Sunflower Seeds	2.0
Whole-wheat Bread	1.6
White Bread	0.2
Oatmeal	1.3
Potato with skin	0.8
Whole Orange	0.5
Orange Juice	0.1
Apple with skin	1.0
Applesauce	0.6
Apple Juice	trace

ITEMS TO AVOID

The following items should be avoided as much as possible from the diet, with allowances, of course, for the occasional splurge. The items to avoid are: refined sugars, red meats, excesssive protein, excessive salt, excessive fat, butter and margarine, soft drinks, alcoholic beverages, coffee and tea, canned and preserved foods, and high cholesterol foods.

Refined Sugar: Our Sweetest Enemy

Avoid or at least significantly reduce the use of white and brown sugars, raw sugar, honey, molasses, syrups, and dextrose. These are, for the most part, "empty calories." Artificial sweeteners such as aspartame (Nutrasweet) and saccharin are not recommended on this dietary program either. Diabetics should check with their physicians and follow their recommendations and guidelines for a healthy diet.

Table VIII-5
HIDDEN SUGARS IN FOODS

Food Item	Size Portion	Approximate Sugar Content in Tsp. Granulated	Food Item	Size Portion	Approximate Sugar Content in Tsp. Granulated
BEVERAGES			*CANDIES*		
Cola drinks	6.0 oz.	3.5	Milk chocolate bar	1	2.5
Cordials	.75 oz.	1.5	Chewing gum	1	0.5
Ginger ale	6.0 oz.	5.0	Fudge	1.0 oz.	4.5
Hi-ball	8.0 oz.	2.5	Gumdrop	1	2.0
Orange ade	8.0 oz.	5.0	Hard candy	4.0 oz.	20.0
Root beer	10.0 oz.	4.5	Lifesavers	1	0.5
Seven-up	6.0 oz.	3.75	Peanut brittle 1.0 oz.	3.5	
Soda pop	8.0 oz.	5.0			
Sweet cider	8.0 oz.	6.0	*CANNED FRUITS AND JUICES*		
Whiskey sour	3.0 oz.	1.5	Canned apricots	4 halves	3.5
CAKES AND COOKIES			Canned fruit juices	4.0 oz.	2.0
			Canned peaches	2 halves	3.5
Angel food	4.0 oz.	7.0	Fruit salad	4.0 oz.	2.5
Applesauce cake	4.0 oz.	5.5	Fruit syrup	2 Tbsp.	2.5
Banana cake	2.0 oz.	2.0	Stewed fruits	4.0 oz.	2.0
Cheesecake	4.0 oz.	2.0			
Chocolate cake (plain)	4.0 oz.	6.0	*DAIRY PRODUCTS*		
Chocolate cake (iced)	4.0 oz.	10.0	Ice cream	3.5 oz.	3.5
Coffeecake	4.0 oz.	4.5	Ice cream bar	1	1-7.0
Cupcake (iced)	4.0 oz.	6.0	Ice cream cone	1	3.5
Fruitcake	4.0 oz.	5.0	Ice cream soda	1	5.0
Jelly-roll	2.0 oz.	2.5	Ice cream sundae	1	7.0
Orange cake	4.0 oz.	4.0	Malted milk shake	10.0 oz.	5.0
Pound cake	4.0 oz.	5.0			
Sponge cake	1.0 oz.	2.0	*JAMS AND JELLIES*		
Strawberry shortcake	1.0 oz.	4.0	Apple butter	1 Tbsp.	1.0
Brownies	.75 oz.	3.0	Jelly	1 Tbsp.	1-1.5
Chocolate cookies	1	1.5	Orange marmalade	1 Tbsp.	1-1.5
Fig Newtons	1	5.0	Peach butter	1 Tbsp.	1.0
Ginger snaps	1	3.0	Strawberry jam	1 Tbsp.	1-1.5
Macaroons	1	6.0			
Nut cookies	1	1.5	*DESSERTS*		
Oatmeal cookies	1	2.0	Apple cobbler	4.0 oz.	3.0
Sugar cookies	1	1.5	Blueberry cobbler	4.0 oz.	3.0
Chocolate eclair	1	7.0	Custard	4.0 oz.	2.0
Cream puff	1	2.0	French pastry	4.0 oz.	5.0
Donut (plain)	1	3.0	Jello	4.0 oz.	4.5
Donut (glazed)	1	6.0			

Reprinted with permission from Kurt W. Donsbach, Ph.D.

If you do have a problem with craving sweets, gradually and progressively substitute fresh fruits for refined sugars whenever necesary. If you decide to splurge on sweets once in a while, it's okay. It's not what you do once in a while, but what you do on a regular basis that's important. I call it the 90/10 program—90 percent of the time you stick to your dietary program, and the other 10 percent you allow yourself a small splurge.

Look at Table VIII-5 to find out approximately how much sugar there is in some of the everyday foods we eat.

Nathan Pritikin, famed founder of the Longevity Center in Santa Monica, points out that: "Table sugar, honey, molasses, and so forth have the property of increasing blood fats (triglycerides) and increasing the clinical signs of diabetes. Diabetes and atherosclerosis are related, because they're caused by certain of the same dietary elements."

Dr. Thomas Jukes, University of California at Berkeley, explains in an article on sugar that: "Those who say white sugar is bad, but brown sugar is good, and honey even better, are mistaken. Brown sugar is basically sucrose coated with molasses. Honey has a different make-up, but the amount of vitamins and minerals it supplies is negligible. Nutritionally speaking, the three products are just about the same."

It is also well known and documented that refined sugars contribute to dental cavities. Minimizing the intake of refined carbohydrates and following good dental hygiene prevents the growth of bacteria that play a role in promoting tooth decay.

Is Sugar a Factor in the Development of Diabetes?

Here, the evidence is conflicting. Some studies indicate that sucrose (table sugar) is a factor in the development of diabetes,[9] while other studies have found no relationship between sugar intake and diabetes.[10] Recent evidence, however, inticates that the traditional advice given to diabetics about eating complex carbohydrates such as rice and potatoes, rather than simple carbohydrates such as sugars like glucose, sucrose, and fructose may be incorrect.[11] Recent research by Phyllis Crapo and her associates at the University of Colorado Health Sciences Center in Denver reveals that previously recommended complex carbohydrates such as bread, corn, and potatoes produce high glucose responses.[12]

For years, complex carbohydrates such as rice, potatoes, and corn have been recommended to diabetics. It was assumed that they took longer to be absorbed and as a result would produce only a moderate rise in blood glucose and insulin. However, research by Crapo has demonstrated that a bowl of ice cream or a sweet potato, for example, does almost nothing to blood glucose levels. Conversely, a white potato or a slice of whole wheat or white bread sends blood glucose soaring.[13] To further complicate matters, the effects of carbohydrates on blood glucose are unpredictable. The bottom line is that foods have to be tested on an individual level to determine their glucose response.

Phyllis Crapo, along with Jerrold Olefsky, a diabetologist also at the University of Colorado, tested rice, corn, bread, and potatoes—the four major starches in the diet of Americans. The glucose responses, in increasing order, were rice, bread, corn, and then potatoes. Olefsky points out that: "Potatoes are like candy as far as a diabetic is concerned."

They tried experiments in people with impaired glucose intolerance and with diabetes. The results were the same. They then tried similar experiments using simple sugars, because as Olefsky explains, "We always were taught that a simple sugar is a simple sugar, but it turns out that simple sugars are as different as potatoes and rice." Lactose and fructose have little effect on blood glucose. Sucrose (table sugar) has a moderate effect. Glucose and maltose give immediate and pronounced effects.

Olefsky believes that the one reason for these differences is because of the differences in the accessibility of the starch in various foods.[14] The more homogenized the food, the more rapid the rise in blood glucose.[15] A rice slurry gives more rise than rice grains. Apple puree gives a more rapid rise than a whole apple.[16]

The whole process of studying the blood-glucose response of foods has been an eye-opener for nutritionists. As Crapo further explains: "What happens when we eat food is much more complex than anyone thought."

If you're diabetic, check with your physician for specific guidelines relating to your individual condition.

Red Meats

This may be one of the most difficult foods for many people to avoid or at least significantly reduce, since we in the Western world are heavy meat eaters. According to the U.S. Department of Agriculture, beef consumption in the United States was 55 pounds per person in 1940, rising to 127 pounds per person in 1977. However, by 1987, it had dropped to only 103 pounds per person and is still dropping. On the other hand, poultry consumption in 1977 was only about 44 pounds per person, and by 1987 it rose to a stately 78 pounds per person—nearly doubling in ten years. During this same period, fish consumption has tripled!

What does all this statistical information tell us? Well, first I want to say that this is not a personal attack on the beef industry. It's merely a recommendation to either avoid or significantly reduce the consumption of red meat.

Unfortunately, there are many people in this nation who are combating diseases such as heart disease, strokes, gallbladder disease, and obesity. Many of these conditions can be directly or partially linked to things such as genetic predisposition, lack of exercise, stress, and a high-fat, high-cholesterol diet. It is for this reason that red meat and other high-fat foods should either be avoided or significantly reduced. See Table VIII-2 for a comparative analysis of red meat to fish and poultry.

Protein

In this country, we seem to have a love affair with protein. Our psyche has been ingrained with phrases like "high-protein drink," "high-protein food," and "high-protein tablets." Protein de-

Table VIII-6 GUIDELINES FOR PROTEIN CONSUMPTION		
Age (years)		*Protein (grams)*
Children	1-3	23
	4-6	30
	7-10	34
Males	11-14	45
	15-18	56
	19-22	56
	23-50	56
	51+	56
Females	11-14	46
	15-18	46
	19-22	44
	23-50	44
	51+	44
Pregnant	-	30 additional
Lactating	-	20 additional

ficiencies such as kwashiorkor and marasmus (protein/calorie deficiency), for example, are virtually unheard of in this country. Moreover, current research indicates that we require considerably less protein than we are led to believe. The report published by the 1980 National Research Council on Food and Nutrition recommends using the guidelines in Table VIII-6.

Although the Luna Diet recommends significant reduction of red meat and limited amounts of fish and poultry, all of which are high in protein, it is still a relatively simple matter to meet your protein requirements. After determining your protein requirements from the chart, the next step is to find out whether you are meeting them. The list of foods and their protein values in Table VIII-7 will assist you in making this determination.

As you can see, it's relatively simple to meet your protein requirements. However, sometimes it's very difficult to convince people of this, because they have been programmed to think that to be healthy one must eat a great deal of protein. Conditions where increased consumption of protein might be justified are kwashiorkor (a protein deficiency), infectious hepatitis, ulcerative colitis, prolonged diarrhea, and anemia.[17] Increased protein consumption is also recommended for hypoglycemia (low blood sugar).[18] Dieticians are also recommending higher amounts of protein for AIDS patients.

Are Large Amounts of Protein Essential to Athletes in Training?

Many of the professional and non-professional athletes whom I counsel are under the impression they require large amounts of

Table VIII-7 PROTEIN VALUES OF COMMON FOODS		
	Amount	*Protein (grams)*
DAIRY PRODUCTS		
Milk (non-fat)	1 cup	9
Milk (low-fat)	1 cup	10
Cottage cheese (low-fat)	1 cup	31
Mozzarella cheese (part skim)	1 oz.	8
Yogurt (low-fat)	1 cup	8
Eggs	1 egg	6
VEGETABLES, NUTS, BEANS AND PEAS		
Almonds (shelled)	1 cup	26
Beans (red kidney)	1 cup	15
Peas (split, dry)	1 cup	20
Peas (green)	1 cup	9
Sunflower seeds	1 cup	24
Broccoli	1 stalk	6
Spinach (cooked)	1 cup	5
Apricots (dried)	1 cup	8
Tomato	1 medium	2
Tofu (soybean curd)	4 oz.	11
GRAIN PRODUCTS		
Rye bread	1 slice	2
Barley (uncooked)	1 cup	16
Oatmeal or rolled oats	1 cup	5
Rice (white, cooked)	1 cup	4
MEAT, POULTRY, AND FISH		
Chicken (broiled)	1/2 breast	20
Ham	3 1/2 oz.	18
Steak (sirloin, broiled)	3 oz.	20
Tuna	3 oz.	23
Turkey (light meat)	3 1/2 oz.	29
Swordfish (broiled)	3 oz.	23

protein. Many feel that strenuous or vigorous physical activity results in protein loss, because of the wear and tear on muscle fiber. However, if this assumption were true, the body, in breaking down protein, which consists of carbon, hydrogen, oxygen, and nitrogen, would excrete nitrogen in the form of urea. Ellington Darden, of the Food and Nutrition Department at Florida State University, points out that numerous experiments on nitrogen balance indicate that the amount of nitrogen the body secretes after vigorous exercise is not significantly higher than the amounts excreted when the body has been resting. He adds that cross-country skiers, for example, who raced from 22 to 53 miles in one day excreted no more nitrogen following this workout than following sleep or rest.[19]

Another interesting study was done by Per-Olof Astrand, M.D., who conducted experiments to determine the best diet for athletes. He gave nine male subjects a mixed diet of protein, fat, and carbohydrates, and found that they could pedal a bicycle 1 hour and 54 minutes before exhaustion. Then, after three days on a diet high in fat and protein including meat, eggs, and milk, the subjects again exercised on the bicycles. This time they pedaled an average of only 57 minutes before becoming exhausted.

Next, the nine participants followed a high complex-carbohydrate diet, such as the Luna Diet, for three days before exercising again on the stationary bicycles. The men were then able to pedal an average of 2 hours and 47 minutes—almost 2 hours longer than before! Some of the men on the complex-carbohydrate diet even managed to continue as long as 4 hours.[20]

It becomes clear on the basis of all these facts that, if a large part of the diet is comprised of animal protein, it would be in your best interests to decrease your total protein intake. Heavy protein consumption is not essential, and red meats are not necessary to make you feel strong. Let's discard this myth once and for all.

The pre-game meal no longer consists of steak. Athletes are now being given complex carbohydrates such as spaghetti, whole-wheat products, potatoes, brown rice, etc., prior to a game or other event to increase glycogen ("reserve fuel") levels. The other advantage is that complex carbohydrates are converted into glycogen more easily than proteins or fats.

Salt: An Acquired Taste

The average American consumes approximately 6 to 18 grams of salt per day (1 teaspoon of salt is about 5 grams).[21] The Luna Diet recommendation is to consume less than 2 grams of salt per day. This amount is safe, and you will find it to be adequate.

Excessive salt may cause fluid retention in some people. In certain conditions, if sodium

Table VIII-8
ENDURANCE COMPARISONS
FOR THREE BASIC DIETS

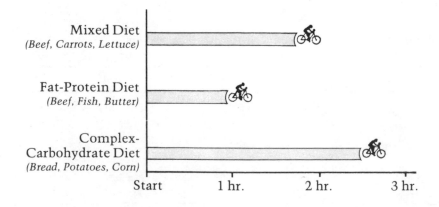

cannot be eliminated, additional water may be held in the body to keep the sodium concentration of the fluid at a constant level. As a result, swelling of the tissues (edema) may result. Most people, however, promptly excrete excess salt no matter how high their dietary intake.

Salt consumption should be watched by people who have kidney disease, high blood pressure, cerebral vascular disease, and heart disease. It may also make a weight-reduction program more difficult, particularly if there is a tendency in the individual to retain water.

Salt is an essential mineral that is necessary for water balance, acid-base balance, nerve-cell activation, muscle contraction, and osmotic pressure. The recommendation therefore is not to eliminate salt in the diet altogether, but rather to reduce your total salt intake as much as possible by slowly re-acclimating your taste buds.

There are numbers of people who sit down to eat and automatically sprinkle salt all over their food before even tasting it. You could start by reducing or eliminating altogether the salt that you normally add to food when cooking or eating. Concurrently, you can reduce your intake of foods that contain large amounts of salt, particularly processed foods.

Are salt tablets ever necessary? Traditionally, the rule of thumb is, if you drink more than 4 quarts of water a day to replace water lost in exercise, you should take a gram of salt (a tablet about the size of an aspirin is equal to a gram) with each additional quart.[22] However, your best option for workouts involving profuse sweating (more than 4 quarts) are electrolyte replacement drinks instead of salt tablets. Otherwise, your best source of hydration is water.

Look at Table VIII-9 to understand what foods have the most sodium and the sodium content of some everyday foods.

A Matter of Fat

In the Luna Diet, the recommendation is to decrease the consumption of all fats as much as possible. Fat tastes great, but an over-consumption of it could be potentially dangerous—even fatal.

The average American eats a diet that contains about 40 percent to 45 percent fat. The Luna Diet recommends a diet that consists of approximately 20% of its total calories from fat. Saturated fats are generally derived from animal sources and are normally solid or firm at room temperature, whereas polyunsaturated fats are from a plant source, and are normally liquid at room temperature. The exceptions include coconut oil, palm kernel oil, and chocolate fat (cocoa butter), all of which have a high percentage of saturated fat.

Fats are not either all saturated or all polyunsaturated. Foods contain a combination of both saturated and polyunsaturated fats, with one or the other dominating.

Also, don't be fooled by foods prepared with hydrogenated vegetable oils. Once a polyunsaturated fat is hydrogenated (artificially hardened), it becomes more saturated.

Saturated fats, when taken in excess, can not only elevate triglycerides (fats in the blood), but may also elevate the amount of cholesterol normally found in the blood. Elevated amounts of cholesterol have been linked to atherosclerotic lesions (fatty deposits in the arteries) that sometimes build up to restrict the flow of blood to the heart. It's this type of blockage that may result in a heart attack or a stroke.

Scientific evidence has shown that polyunsaturated fats are *not* necessarily safer than saturated fats. Dr. Meyer Friedman and his associates in San Francisco demonstrated that unsaturated fats in the diet produced just as much fat blockage in the capillaries as ordinary animal fat and often stayed in the bloodstream longer!

One of Dr. Friedman's studies, documented in the *Journal of the American Medical Association,* involved forty firemen from San Francisco. To determine blockages, photographs were taken of the capillaries in the subjects' eyes. Before the subjects had anything to eat or drink, the vessels were open, showing no blockage. Dr. Friedman then gave each of the subjects a glass of heavy cream. Five hours after the heavy cream drink, approximately twenty-five blockages were found in the subjects' eyes. Later, after the blood vessels had cleared, they were given safflower oil, a polyunsaturated fat. Five hours after the oil drink, there were just as many blockages of the same severity as after the cream drink. Dr.

Table VIII-9
SODIUM CONTENT OF COMMON FOODS

TABLE SALTS

PLAIN SALT: 100% sodium chloride
IODIZED SALT: 100% sodium chloride with iodine added
LIGHT SALT: 50% sodium chloride and 50% potassium chloride.
SALT SUBSTITUTE: 100% potassium chloride. Large amounts of potassium chloride may cause irregular heart beats. Do not use without consulting your doctor.

FOODS HIGH IN SALT (SODIUM)

MEAT, MEAT FLAVORINGS, AND FISH

Anchovies	Dried Cod	Meat tenderizers
Bacon	Frankfurters	Salted and smoked fish
Bacon fat	Ham	Salted and smoked meats
Canned meat	Herring	Sardines
Caviar	Luncheon meats	Sausages
Corned beef	Meat extracts and sauces	Tuna (in oil)

APPETIZERS, SAUCES, AND SEASONINGS

Cheeses	Olives	Relishes
Celery salt	Onion salt	Salted nuts
Chili sauce	Pickles	Salted popcorn
Garlic salt	Potato chips	Sauerkraut
Ketchup	Pretzels	Soy sauce
Mustard	Regular bouillon cubes	Table salt
		Worcestershire sauce

FOODS MODERATELY HIGH IN SALT (SODIUM)

BREADS AND CEREALS

Breads	Crackers	Waffles
Corn flakes	Rolls	

VEGETABLES

Canned vegetables	Canned vegetable juices	Celery

DAIRY PRODUCTS

Cheese	Salted butter	Salted margarine

MEAT AND FISH

Clams	Kidneys	Oysters
Crabs	Lobsters	Scallops
		Shrimp

OTHER ITEMS

Baking powder	Beverage mixes	Molasses
		Salad dressings

SODIUM AND POTASSIUM CONTENT IN FOODS

MEAT AND POULTRY	Portion	Sodium (mg)	Potassium (mg)	Calories
BACON	1 strip	71	16	156
BEEF				
Corned Beef (canned)	3 slices	803	51	184
Hamburger	3/4 lb.	41	382	224
Pot Roast (rump)	1/2 lb.	43	309	188
Sirloin Steak	1/2 lb.	57	545	260
CHICKEN				
Broiler	3 1/2 oz.	78	320	151
DUCK	3 1/2 oz.	82	285	326
FRANKFURTER	1/8 lb.	550	110	129
HAM				
Fresh	1/4 lb.	37	260	126
Cured, butt	1/4 lb.	518	239	123
Cured, shank	1/4 lb.	336	155	91
LAMB				
Shoulder chop	1/2 lb.	72	422	260
Rib chop	1/2 lb.	68	398	238
Leg roast	1/4 lb.	41	246	96
LIVER				
Beef	3 1/2 oz.	86	325	136
Calf	3 1/2 oz.	131	436	141
PORK				
Loin chop	6 oz.	52	500	314
Spareribs (3 or 4)	3 1/2 oz.	51	360	209
Sausage	3 1/2 oz.	740	140	450
TURKEY	3 1/2 oz.	40	320	268
VEAL				
Cutlet	6 oz.	46	448	235
Loin chop	1/2 lb.	54	384	514
Rump roast	1/4 lb.	36	244	84
FISH				
Clams (4 lg./9 sm.)	3 1/2 oz.	36	235	82
Cod	3 1/2 oz.	70	382	78
Flounder or Sole	3 1/2 oz.	56	366	68
Lobster (broiled with 2 tbsp. butter)	3/4 lb.	210	180	308
Oysters (5-8)	3 1/2 oz.	73	121	66
Salmon (pink/canned)	3 1/2 oz.	387	361	141
Sardines (8)(in oil)	3 1/2 oz.	510	560	311
Shrimp	3 1/2 oz.	140	220	91
Tuna (in oil)	3 1/2 oz.	800	301	288
Tuna (in water)	3 1/2 oz.	41	279	127
SNACKS				
Chocolate creams	1 candy	1	15	51

Milk chocolate	1 oz.	30	105	152
Ice cream				
Chocolate	1/2 pint	75	—	300
Vanilla	1/2 pint	82	210	290
Nuts				
Cashews (roasted)	6-8	2	84	84
Peanuts (roasted)				
Salted	1 Tbsp.	69	105	85
Unsalted	1 Tbsp.	trace	111	86
Olives				
Green	2 medium	312	7	15
Ripe	2 large	150	5	37
Potato chips	5 chips	34	88	54
Pretzels (3 ring)	1 average	87	7	12
DAIRY PRODUCTS				
Butter (salted)	1 pat	99	2	72
Butter (unsalted)	1 pat	01	2	72
Cheese				
American, cheddar	1 oz.	197	23	112
American, processed	1 oz.	318	22	107
Cottage, creamed	3 1/2 oz.	229	85	106
Cream (heavy)	1 Tbsp.	35	10	52
Egg	1 large	66	70	88
Milk (whole)	8 oz.	122	352	159
Margarine (salted)	1 pat	99	2	72
BREADS AND CEREALS				
Rye	1 slice	128	33	56
White (enriched)	1 slice	117	20	62
Whole wheat	1 slice	121	63	56
Corn Flakes	1 cup	165	40	95
Macaroni (enriched)	1 cup	1	85	151
Noodles (enriched)	1 cup	3	70	200
Oatmeal	1 cup	1	130	148
Rice (white, dry)	1/4 cup	3	45	178
Spaghetti (enriched)	1 cup	2	92	166
Waffles (enriched)	1 waffle	356	109	209
Wheat germ	3 Tbsp.	1	232	102
BEVERAGES				
Apple juice	6 oz.	2	187	87
Beer	8 oz.	8	46	114
Coca-Cola	6 oz.	2	88	78
Coffee	1 cup	3	149	5
Cranberry cocktail	7 oz.	2	20	130
Ginger ale	8 oz.	18	1	80
Orange juice (canned)	8 oz.	3	500	120
Prune juice	6 oz.	4	423	138
Tea	8 oz.	2	21	2

FRUITS				
Apple	1 medium	1	165	87
Apricot				
Fresh	2-3	1	281	51
Canned (in syrup)	3 halves	1	234	86
Dried	17 halves	26	979	260
Banana	1 whole	1	370	85
Blueberries	1 cup	1	81	62
Cantaloupe	1/4 melon	12	251	30
Cherries				
Fresh	1/2 cup	2	191	58
Canned (in syrup)	1/2 cup	1	124	89
Dates				
Fresh	10 medium	1	648	274
Dried	1 cup (6 oz.)	2	1150	488
Fruit cocktail	1/2 cup	5	161	76
Grapefruit	1/2 medium	1	135	41
Grapes	22 grapes	3	158	69
Orange	1 small	1	200	49
Peaches				
Fresh	1 medium	1	202	38
Canned	2 halves			
(in syrup)		2	130	78
Pears				
Fresh	1/2 pear	2	130	61
Canned	2 halves			
(in syrup)		1	84	76
Pineapple				
Fresh	3/4 cup	1	146	52
Canned	1 slice (in syrup)	1	96	74
Plums				
Fresh	2 medium	2	299	66
Canned	3 medium			
(in syrup)		1	142	83
Prunes, dried	10 large	8	694	255
Strawberries	10 large	1	164	37
Watermelon	1/2 cup	1	100	26
VEGETABLES				
Artichoke	1 large bud	30	301	44
Asparagus				
Fresh	2/3 cup	1	183	20
Canned	6 spears	271	191	21
Beans, baked	5/8 cup	2	704	159
Beans, green				
Fresh	1 cup	5	189	31
Canned	1 cup	295	109	30
Beans, lima				
Fresh	5/8 cup	1	422	111

Canned	1/2 cup	271	255	110
Frozen	5/8 cup	129	394	118
Beets				
Fresh	1/2 cup	36	172	27
Canned	1/2 cup	196	138	31
Broccoli, fresh	2/3 cup	10	267	26
Brussels sprouts	6-7 medium	10	273	36
Cabbage				
Raw, shredded	1 cup	20	233	24
Cooked	3/5 cup	14	163	20
Carrots				
Raw	1 large	47	341	42
Cooked	2/3 cup	33	222	31
Canned	2/3 cup	236	120	30
Cauliflower	7/8 cup	9	206	22
Celery	4 stalks	63	170	8
Corn				
Fresh	1 ear	trace	196	100
Canned	1/2 cup	196	81	70
Cucumber, pared	1/2 medium	3	80	7
Lettuce, iceberg	3 1/2 oz.	9	264	14
Mushrooms	10 sm./4 lg.	15	414	28
Onions	1 medium	10	157	38
Peas				
Fresh	2/3 cup	1	196	71
Canned	3/4 cup	236	96	88
Frozen	3 1/2 oz.	115	135	68
Potatoes				
Boiled	1 medium	3	407	76
French fried	10 pieces	3	427	137
Radishes	10 small	18	322	17
Sauerkraut	2/3 cup	747	140	18
Spinach	1/2 cup	45	291	21
Tomatoes				
Raw	1 medium	4	366	33
Canned	1/2 cup	130	217	21

*All Portions weigh 3½ oz. unless otherwise noted.

Source: *C.F. Church and H.N. Church,* Food Values of Portions Commonly Used, *llth ed. (Philadelphia: J.B. Lippincott Company), 1970.*

Friedman's conclusion was that substituting polyunsaturated fats for saturated fats is not the solution to the problem of blood vessel blockage, since both block the capillaries of the eye. So he urged reduction of *all* fats in the diet.[23]

In another study, Dr. Marvin Bierenbaum and his associates in New Jersey performed a similar experiment with 200 men who had already had heart attacks. The results showed that unsaturated fats are no better at alleviating the risks of subsequent heart attacks than saturated fats.[24]

Another reason for decreasing fat in the diet is due to the calories-per-gram ratio. Look at the Table VIII-10.

You receive almost three times more calories

from fat than from carbohydrates and protein!

To calculate a food's percentage of calories from fat, do the following:

1. Check the product label for grams of fat in one serving. Also check for the number of calories per serving.
2. Multiply the number of fat grams by 10 (fat contains between 9-11 calories per gram). This will give you the number of calories from fat.
3. Divide the number of calories from fat by the number of calories in a serving. For example, if a food contains 130 calories per serving and contains 8 grams of fat, multiply the 8 grams of fat by 10. This gives you 80. Then divide 80 by 130 (calories per serving).

$$80 \div 130 = .61$$

This tells you that this particular food yields 61% of its calories from fat, which needless to say, is too high. Also, don't waste time reading what a product has on the front label (Lite, Healthy, Dietetic, etc.), which in many cases is deceptive. Instead, look for the list of ingredients to see what it contains and then calculate to determine how much of it is fat.

Table VIII-10 CALORIES PER GRAM RATIOS	
Carbohydrates =	4 calories per gram
Protein =	4 calories per gram
Fat =	9-11 calories per gram*

Karen Donato, D.M. Hegsted, "Efficiency of Utilization of Various Sources of Energy for Growth," Proceedings of the National Academy of Sciences, Vol. 82, p.p. 4866-4870, August 1985.

Butter and Margarine

If I had to select 10 of the most useless and counterproductive products ever developed for human consumption, butter and margarine would be close to the top of the list. One pat of butter or margarine consist of 100% fat.

Frequently, I'm asked, "Which is better, margarine or butter? I was under the impression that margarine was better than butter because it has no cholesterol and is lower in saturated fat. Now I'm getting conflicting reports. Who's right?"

Well, this is certainly not an easy question to answer at this time, due primarily to insufficient evidence. Much of the controversy centers around the hydrogenation process (artificial hardening of vegetable fat) that margarine goes through to give it its solid form. One of the recent reports indicates that a certain number of the fatty acids in margarine take on a form that is generally not found in nature.[25] There is not yet any evidence to show that these fatty acids are harmful, but they are incorporated into the cellular walls, and research into their possible toxicity is presently underway.[26]

It is also interesting to note that margarines vary in their degree of saturation. Some are as saturated as butter.

The recommendation is to eliminate or decrease the consumption of both butter and margarine as much as possible from your diet. This becomes particularly important if you have a weight problem, a vascular or heart condition, gall bladder disease, or elevated cholesterol or triglycerides. If you must have an occasional pat of butter or margarine, it's no big deal. Otherwise, avoid the stuff. The use of butter or margarine, as with salt, is an acquired taste, not a required one.

Fried Foods

Avoid fried foods. They not only increase caloric content, but also increase fat content. Steam, broil, or bake foods.

Salad Dressings

Avoid rich salad dressings such as Roquefort, Blue Cheese, French, Thousand Island, and mayonnaise. Of all the dressings mentioned, mayonnaise is the highest in fat and calories. Use either lemon juice, apple cider vinegar, Spike seasoning, or an herb dressing.

Soft Drinks (Sweetened/Carbonated)

Avoid soft drinks. They contain too much sugar and too many empty calories. Some soft drinks also contain saccharin, caffeine, and artificial colors and flavors. The following is a list of the ingredients found in some popular soft drinks:

Diet Pepsi (Sugar Free)

carbonated water	sodium citrate
caramel color	caffeine
phosphoric acid	natural flavors
sodium saccharin	citric acid

Diet Shasta

carbonated water	gum arabic
citric acid	artificial flavor
sodium saccharin	salt
artificial color	saccharin

preserved with erythorbic acid and less than 1 percent sodium benzoate

Alcoholic Beverages

The problems associated with alcohol are known and well documented. I realize there's a world of difference between the occasional social drinker and a chronic alcoholic. However, any substance that may cause liver or kidney disease, weight gain, and psychological and physical addiction is not a part of this program.

Coffee and Tea

Whenever possible, replace regular tea with herb teas and regular coffee with decaffeinated coffee. The purpose is obvious—decrease caffeine consumption. Caffeine is not recommended for the following reasons: (a) There is evidence that caffeine ingested daily over a long period of time increases an individual's susceptibility to coronary artery disease by increasing free fatty acids through central nervous system stimulation.[27] (b) Caffeine may cause complications in delivery.[28] (c) Caffeine increases gastric (stomach) secretions that may eventually induce ulcers in susceptible individuals.[29]

Which has more caffeine—coffee or tea? Ounce per ounce, dry tea has more caffeine than dry coffee. However, we have to keep in mind that it takes more dry ingredient to make a cup of coffee than it does to make a cup of tea. Therefore, if we're measuring both substances in liquid form, one cup of coffee would contain more. But, if the measurements are made in dry form, ounce per ounce, tea contains more caffeine.

Along with tea and coffee, caffeine is also contained in the following items: diet pills, headache remedies, cold and allergy pills, and soft drinks. Table VIII-11 will give you an idea of the caffeine content in some popular soft drinks.

Foods with Many Preservatives

Foods with long lists or preservatives should be avoided whenever possible. They generally contain too many additives, salt, and sugar. In many cases, the nutritional value is inferior to fresh foods. Convenience foods such as frozen

Table VIII-11 SOFT DRINKS WITH CAFFEINE	
(Milligrams per 12-ounce can)	
Diet Rite	36
RC Cola	36
Pepsi Light	36
Diet Pepsi	36
Pepsi-Cola	38
Dr. Pepper	40
Mr. Pibb	40
Sunkist Orange	40
Shasta Diet Cola	44
Shasta Cherry Cola	44
Coca-Cola	45
Tab	46
Mountain Dew	54
Sugar-Free Mr. Pibb	60

Canada Dry Ginger Ale, Hire's Root Beer, Fresca, Fanta soft drinks, Teem, 7-Up, and RC 100 are caffeine free, according to *Good Health Digest* (July, 1982). For comparison, a 5-ounce cup of coffee contains 100-120 mgs. of caffeine.

TV dinners, for example, should be avoided. If you haven't gotten into the habit of doing so, start taking a closer look at the labels of the foods you buy. See Chapter 9 on ingredients and additives.

Cholesterol

There have been innumerable investigations and epidemiological studies performed linking elevated cholesterol levels with coronary artery disease. The recommendation for decrease in the consumption of foods that are high in cholesterol and fat is based on the results of these investigations.

Cholesterol is a fat-like chemical (sterol). It can be made by the body (manufactured by the liver) or can be obtained in the foods we eat. Some of the functions of cholesterol are: (1) it's converted into bile acids, which are necessary for the digestion of fats; (2) it's important in the metabolism of various steroid hormones, such as sex hormones; and (3) it's a part of every cell.

Foods that have the highest cholesterol content are organ meats (liver, brains, kidneys), egg yolks, dairy products, and shellfish.

The recommendation made by the World Health Organization is to maintain your serum cholesterol level below 200 mg.[30] The Luna Diet recommendation is to keep your cholesterol below 160 mg. If your family has a history of heart disease and you don't know what your cholesterol level is, request a lipid profile (blood test that measures cholesterol and other fats in the blood).

Table VIII-12 gives an example of some average ranges of total plasma cholesterol levels in Americans today.[31]

The lipid profile also consists of a check on high-density lipoproteins (HDL), low-density lipoproteins (LDL), and triglycerides (a type of fat).

Lipoproteins are substances that carry cholesterol in the blood. The HDLs are the "good guys" and the LDLs are the "bad guys." HDL cholesterol has been found to be the best serum predictor of coronary artery disease. High levels of the HDL are associated with low risk of coronary artery disease, and conversely low levels with a high risk.[32] HDL appears to be the cholesterol "scavenger" in the body. It removes cholesterol from cells and carries it to the liver for excretion. On the other hand, LDL links up with receptors on cellular surfaces and delivers cholesterol into the cells.

To determine your HDL ratio, simply divide your cholesterol level by your HDL. For example, if your cholesteral level is 220 mg. and your HDL is 65, your HDL ratio is 3.3, which puts you in the low risk category. The Scripp's Clinic HDL ratios from La Jolla, California are provided in Table VIII-13.

Recently, I met a woman who was admitted into the hospital for coronary bypass surgery. Her cholesterol level since childhood has been in the 600-700 mg. range, which is extremely high. She's now in her early forties. Dietary intervention and increases in physical activity were helpful, but not significantly in her particular case. Diagnosis: genetically elevated cholesterol level (type II hyperlipoproteinemia). Cause: Liver receptor deficiency. So why wouldn't a low-cholesterol

Table VIII-12
AVERAGE PLASMA CHOLESTEROL LEVELS IN THE U.S.*

Age	Men mg%	Women mg%
20	166	164
30	192	175
40	206	193
50	213	218
60	213	231
70	208	228

*Source: David Blankenhorn, M.D., "Regression of Atherosclerosis—Integration of Diet and Drugs," American Heart Association Seminar, L.A. Orthopedic Hospital, June 4, 1985.

Table VIII-13
SCRIPPS CLINIC HDL RATIOS

<3.5	=	low risk
3.5 - 5	=	moderate risk
>5	=	high risk

diet solve the problem? Sometimes lipid regulation is not as simplistic as it may appear on the surface. We are all born with a certain number of liver receptors, which determine and regulate serum cholesterol. If the number of liver receptors is low at birth or the number declines with age, total plasma cholesterol levels remain high and relatively unsteady. The treatment for the woman in question will generally consist of drugs such as cholestipol or cholestyramine, in conjunction with a low-cholesterol diet.

The reason for pointing out this particular case is because many of the people we see are under the impression that their serum cholesterol is dependent upon the amount of fat and cholesterol consumed in the diet. Dietary cholesterol is obviously a relevant factor, but it only accounts for about 25 percent of the total cholesterol in your body. The other 75 percent is produced by the body. This does not mean that the restriction of dietary cholesterol isn't important, but only that the body itself already produces a large proportion of this substance. *The amount of cholesterol in the body at any one time not only depends on dietary intake, but on the percentage of absorption, endogenous (internal) cholesterol synthesis, transport from one location in the body to another, conversion to bile acids, and excretion.*

One other thing to keep in mind is that you can have twelve people on the same identical diet and still have twelve different levels of cholesterol.

Dr. Charles Glueck, Director of the Lipo-protein and Lipid Research Clinic at the University of Cincinnati College of Medicine, explains that about 85 percent of adults under age 50 who have had a heart attack have an elevated total cholesterol and/or triglyceride level or low levels of high density lipoproteins.[33]

Another study done at the Cleveland Clinic in Cleveland, Ohio, involving 723 young men with slight chest pain found that elevated cholesterol levels were correlated to significant artery closure. Table VIII-14 shows the results of the study.[34]

Dr. David Blankenhorn, of the USC School of Medicine, points out that the average man or woman in this country who has a coronary bypass also has a cholesterol level averaging in the 265 mg. range. If the patient smokes, has high blood pressure, is obese, and doesn't exercise, the risk factors increase significantly.

Investigators are finding that atherosclerosis (degenerative blockage of an artery) begins at a very early age in the United States. Fatty streaks, for example, have been observed in the aortas of infants less than a year old.[35] Dr. William Castelli (Director of the Framingham Study) recently pointed out that three-fourths of American teenagers start forming artery lesions during their teens. During the Korean and Vietnam wars, many men in their early twenties were killed. In both of these wars, several studies were performed on the hearts of hundreds of these young soldiers killed in battle to see how wide-spread heart disease was among American soldiers.

One study reported in the *Journal of the American Medical Association* involved 300 soldiers killed in Korea. The average age of these soldiers was 22 years. Of the autopsies performed on these men, more than 50 percent had artery damage from plaques formed in the coronary arteries. A comparative study on Koreans also killed in the war showed virtually no evidence of this disease.[36]

In another study involving more than 100 soldiers killed in South Vietnam, 50 percent of the autopsies showed normal coronary arteries, 45 percent had medium artery damage, and 5 percent had severe artery damage. The average age of these soldiers was also about 22 years.[37]

The Luna Diet recommendations to help you

Table VIII-14
CORRELATION OF CHOLESTEROL LEVELS TO SIGNIFICANT ARTERY CLOSURE

Cholesterol Level	% of Significant Artery Closure
Less than 200	20
201-225	38
226-250	48
251-275	60
276-300	77
301-350	80
More than 350	91

reduce your cholesterol are as follows:

1. Decrease all dietary fats (saturated, polyunsaturated, monosaturated, etc.)
2. Decrease cholesterol intake to 100 mg. per 1,000 calories ingested
3. Maintain serum cholesterol level below 160 mg.

4. Avoid smoking or inhaling passive smoke (it tends to depress HDL levels)
5. Exercise (preferably 20 minutes of aerobic activity three times per week)
6. Achieve and maintain an ideal body weight

Table VIII-15 provides a list of foods and their approximate cholesterol content.

Table VIII-15
CHOLESTEROL CONTENT OF FOODS*

Approximate Amounts of Cholesterol in Milligrams Per 100 Gram (3 1/2 oz) Portions of Foods

BEEF		*BEEF TALLOW*	56	Haddock	64		
Rump roast	58	*LARD*	65	Codfish	46		
Round steak	68	*CHEESES*		Mackerel	80		
Chuck roast	55	Limburger	92	Herring	75		
Veal	71	Roquefort	73	Perch	63		
PORK		Cream	140	Pike	71		
Chops	55	American		*SHELLFISH*	161		
Tenderloin	57	Process	87	Shrimp	99		
Ham	42	Cheddar	98	Crab	150		
LAMB		Bleu	157	Lobster	50		
Chops	66	Mozzarella	61	Oysters	50		
Mutton	77	(part skim)		Clams	50		
		Swiss	91	Scallops	50		
TURKEY		Gouda	33	*MILK*			
Light	61	Hoop	1	Whole	14		
Dark	96	Parmesan	74	Skim	<1		
CHICKEN		American	92	Buttermilk	6		
Light	54	*FISH*		Butter	249		
Dark	76	Trout	57	*CREAM*			
KIDNEY	300	Tuna	51	Thick	140		
LIVER, BEEF	320	Salmon	55	Thin	40		
BRAINS, CALF	1810	Halibut	33	*SWEET BREADS*	280		

Amounts of Cholesterol in Milligrams Per Serving of Food

1 cup fortified skim milk (less than 1% buttermilk fat)	12	1/2 cup ice milk	17	Peanut butter	0
		1 egg yolk	240	Fruits	0
		1 tsp. butter	10	Vegetables	0
		1 Tbsp. mayonnaise	15	Egg whites	0
1 cup skim milk	1			Cereals	0
1/2 cup sherbet	3	1 Tbsp. thick cream	18	Vegetable oil	0
1 cup whole milk	35				
1/2 cup ice cream	30	Margarine	0		

**From* Low Cholesterol Diet Manual, *Department of Internal Medicine, University of Iowa.*

CHAPTER 8 NOTES

[1] Glasser, William, *Positive Addiction* (New York: Harper & Row, 1976) pp. 4-5.

[2] "Crude Fiber: Questions and Answers," *Modern Medicine,* September 6, 1977.

[3] *Ibid.*

[4] "Roughage in the Diet," *Medical World News,* September 6, 1974, pp. 35-42.

[5] McNaughton, Robert A., *Current Therapy,* (Philadelphia: W.B. Saunders Co., 1980) p. 343.

[6] "Roughage in the Diet," *Medical World News,* September 6, 1974, pp. 35-42.

[7] *Ibid.*

[8] Anastasio, Patricia, "New Ways to Control and Manage Diabetes," *Environmental Nutrition Newsletter,* Volume 5, No. 12, December 1982, p. 1.

[9] Cohen, A. M., *Dietary Sugar and Disease* (Washington, D.C.: Government Printing Office, 1973) p. 167-198.

[10] West, K. M., *Prevention and Therapy of Diabetes Mellitus, Nutrition Reviews' Present Knowledge in Nutrition,* 4th ed. (Washington, D.C.: Nutrition Foundation, 1976) pp. 356-364.

[11] Kolata, G., "Dietary Dogma Disproved," *Science,* Vol. 220, No. 4596, April 29, 1983, pp. 487-88.

[12] *Ibid.*

[13] *Ibid.*

[14] Kolata, G., "Dietary Dogma Disproved," *Science,* Vol. 220, No. 4596, April 29, 1983, pp. 487-88.

[15] *Ibid.*

[16] *Ibid.*

[17] Robinson, Corinne H., *Basic Nutrition and Diet Therapy* (New York: Macmillan Co., 1970) pp. 196-7.

[18] Hamilton, Eva, and Whitney, Eleanor, *Nutrition Concepts and Controversies* (St. Paul: West Publishing Co., 1979) p. 65

[19] Hedman, R., "The Available Glycogen in Man and the Connection Between Rate of Oxygen Intake and Carbohydrate Usage," *Acta Physiology Scandinavia,* Vol. 40, 1957, pp. 305-9.

[20] Astrand, Per-Olof, "Something Old and Something New...Very New," *Nutrition Today,* 1968, p. 9.

[21] *Dietary Goals for the United States, 2nd edition,* (Washington, D.C.: Government Printing Office, 1977) p. 49.

[22] Whitney, E.N., and Hamilton, E.M., *Understanding Nutrition,* (St. Paul: West Publishing Co. 1977) pp. 437-8.

[23] Friedman, Meyer, *et al.,* "The Effect of Unsaturated Fats Upon Lipemia and Conjunctival Circulation," *Journal of American Medical Association,* Vol. 193, 1965, p. 882.

[24] Bierenbaum, Marvin, *et al.,* "The Five Year Experience of Modified Fat Diets on Younger Men with Coronary Heart Disease," *Circulation* 42, 1970, p. 943.

[25] "Questions from Our Readers," *Environmental Nutrition Newsletter,* Vol. 4, No. 5, June 1981.

[26] *Ibid.*

[27] Bellet, Samuel, "Response of Free Fatty Acids to Coffee and Caffeine," *Metabolism,* Vol. 17, 1968, pp. 702-708.

[28] Hamilton, Eva May, and Eleanor Whitney, *Nutrition Concepts and Controversies* (New York: West Punblishing Co., 1979), p. 381.

[29] MacMahon, Brian, Stella Yen, Dimitrios Trichopoulos, and Kenneth Warren, "Coffee and Cancer of the Pancreas," *New England Journal of Medicine,* Vol. 304, March 12, 1981, pp. 630-633.

[30] "Prevention of Coronary Heart Disease," *World Health Organization Report,* Tech. Rep. Ser, WHO, No. 678, 1982.

[31] Blankenhorn, David, M.D., "Regression of Atherosclerosis—Integration of Diet and Drugs", *Americn Heart Association Seminar,* Los Angeles, Orthopedic Hospital, June 4, 1985.

[32] Hooper, et al., "Terbutaline Raises High-Density Lipoprotein Cholesterol Levels," *New England Journal of Medicine,* December 10, 1981, pp. 1455-6.

[33] Gluech, Charles, "Hyperlipidemia," *Diagnosis,* February 1981, p. 80.

[34] Welch, C.C., "Cinecoronary Arteriography in Young Men," *Circulation,* Vol. 62, 1970, p. 625.

[35] Holman, R.L., *et al.,* "The Natural History of Atherosclerosis: The Early Aortic Lesions as seen in New Orleans in the Middle of the 20th Century," *American Journal of Pathology,* 34, 1958, pp. 209-234.

[36] Enos, W.F., et al., "Pathogenesis of Coronary Disease in American Soldiers Killed in Korea," *Journal of the American Medical Association,* July 16, 1955.

[37] McNamara, J.J., et al., "Coronary Artery Disease in Vietnam Casualties," *Journal of the American Medical Association,* Vol. 216, May 17, 1971, pp. 1185-1187.

Chapter 9

INGREDIENTS AND ADDITIVES

A nutritionally oriented person should be aware that labels don't always tell the full story. There are no legal requirements that the actual amounts of various ingredients in food products be given. They are required to be listed in decreasing order of amount. For example, if there is more sugar than grain contained in a box of cereal, the sugar must be listed first.

Many food companies will often combine the grains and split the sugar content by listing each type separately. This way sugar seldom appears as the first ingredient. They will list table sugar, brown sugar, dextrose, molasses, and honey separately, knowing full well that there is not a great deal of difference in the way our bodies receive them.

There are over 2,700 food additives being used in foods. Some of these additives are harmful, and some are not. As a general rule, try to avoid foods with long lists of preservatives. Also keep in mind that the wider the variety of foods that you eat, the greater will be the variety of different chemical substances consumed, thus reducing the chance that any one chemical will reach a hazardous level. This is assuming, of course, that you don't try to subsist on a diet of hot dogs, soft drinks, potato chips, and maraschino cherries.

The following "Chemical Cuisine" information has been reprinted with permission from the Center for Science in the Public Interest in Washington, D.C. It is broken down into three categories: those chemicals that are safe, those that should be used with caution, and those that should be avoided.

SAFE

The following additives appear to be safe:

Alginate, Propylene Glycol Alginate

Function: Thickening agents, foam stabilizer.
Used in: Ice cream, cheese, candy, yogurt

Alginate, an apparently safe derivative of seaweed (kelp), maintains the desired texture in dairy products, canned frosting, and other factory-made foods.

Propylene glycol alginate, a chemically-modified algin, thickens acidic foods (soda pop, salad dressing) and stabilizes the foam in beer.

Alpha Tocopherol (Vitamin E)

Function: Antioxidant, nutrient.
Used in: Vegetable oils.

Vitamin E is abundant in whole wheat, rice germ, and vegetable oils. It is destroyed by the refining and bleaching of flour. Vitamin E prevents oils from going rancid.

Ascorbic Acid (Vitamin C)

Function: Antioxidant, nutrient, color stabilizer.
Used in: Oily foods, cereals, soft drinks, and cured meats.

Ascorbic acid helps maintain the red color of cured meat and prevents the formation of nitrosamines (see sodium nitrate). It helps prevent loss of color and flavor by reacting with unwanted oxygen. It is used as a nutrient additive in drinks and breakfast cereals. Sodium ascorbate is a more soluble form of ascorbic acid. Erythorbic acid serves the same functions as ascorbic acid but has no value as a vitamin.

Beta Carotene

Function: Coloring, nutrient.
Used in: Margarine, shortening, non-dairy whiteners, butter.

Beta carotene is used as an artifical coloring and a nutrient supplement. The body converts it to Vitamin A, which is part of the light-detection mechanism of the eye.

Calcium (or Sodium) Propionate

Function: Preservative.
Used in: Bread, rolls, pies, cakes.

Calcium propionate prevents mold growth on bread and rolls. The calcium is a beneficial mineral; the propionate is safe. Sodium propionate is used in pies and cakes, because calcium alters the action of chemical leavening agents.

Calcium (or Sodium) Stearoyl Lactylate

Function: Dough conditioner, whipping agent.
Used in: Bread dough, cake fillings, artificial whipped cream, processed egg whites.

These additives strengthen bread dough so it can be used in bread-making machinery and lead to more uniform grain and greater volume. They act as whipping agents in dried, liquid, or frozen egg whites and artificial whipped cream. Sodium stearoyl fumarate serves the same function.

Carrageenan

Function: Thickening and stabilizing agent.
Used in: Ice cream, jelly, chocolate milk, infant formula.

Obtained from "Irish Moss" seaweed, it is used as a thickening agent and to stabilize oil-water mixtures.

Casein, Sodium Caseinate

Function: Thickening and whitening agent.
Used in: Ice cream, ice milk, sherbet, coffee creamers.

Casein, the principal protein in milk, is a nutritious protein containing adequate amounts of all the essential amino acids.

Citric Acid, Sodium Citrate

Function: Acid, flavoring, chelating agent.
Used in: Ice cream, sherbet, fruit drink, candy, carbonated beverages, instant potatoes.

Citric acid is versatile, widely used, cheap, and safe. It is an important metabolite in virtually all living organisms, especially abundant in citrus fruits and berries. It is used as a strong acid, a tart flavoring, and an antioxidant. Sodium citrate, also safe, is a buffer that controls the acidity of gelatin deserts, jam, ice cream, candy, and other foods.

EDTA

Function: Chelating agent.
Used in: Salad dressing, margarine, sandwich spreads, mayonnaise, processed fruits and vegetables, canned shellfish, soft drinks.

Modern food manufacturing technology, which involves metal rollers, blenders, and containers, results in trace amounts of metal contamination in food. EDTA (ethylene-diamine tetra acetic acid) traps metal impurities, which would otherwise promote rancidity and the breakdown of artificial colors.

Ferrous Gluconate

Function: Coloring, nutrient.
Used in: Black olives.

Used by the olive industry to generate a uniform jet-black color and in pills as a source of iron. Safe.

Fumaric Acid

Function: Tartness agent.
Used in: Powdered drinks, pudding, pie fillings, gelatin desserts.

A solid at room temperature, inexpensive, highly acidic, it is the ideal source of tartness and acidity in dry food products. However, it dissolves slowly in cold water, a drawback cured by adding dioctyl sodium sulfosuccinate (DSS), a poorly tested, detergent-like additive.

Gelatin

Function: Thickening and gelling agent.
Used in: Powdered dessert mix, yogurt, ice cream, cheese spreads, beverages.

Gelatin is a protein obtained from animal bones, hooves, and other parts. It has little nutritional value, because it contains little or none of several essential amino acids.

Glycerin or Glycerol

Function: Maintains water content.
Used in: Marshmallow, candy, fudge, baked goods.

Glycerin forms the backbone of fat and oil molecules and is quite safe. The body uses it as a source of energy or as a starting material in making more complex molecules.

Hydrolyzed Vegetable Protein (HVP)

Function: Flavor enhancer.

Used in: Instant soups, frankfurters, sauce mixes, beef stew.

HVP consists of vegetable (usually soybean) protein that has been chemically broken down to the amino acids of which it is composed. HVP is used to bring out the natural flavor of food (and perhaps to use less real food).

Lactic Acid

Function: Acidity regulator.
Used in: Spanish olives, cheese, frozen desserts, carbonated beverages.

This safe acid occurs in almost all living organisms. It inhibits spoilage in Spanish-type olives, balances the acidity in cheese-making, and adds tartness to frozen desserts, carbonated fruit-flavored drinks, and other foods.

Lactose

Function: Sweetener.
Used in: Whipped topping mix, breakfast pastry.

Lactose, a carbohydrate found only in milk, is nature's way of delivering calories to infant mammals. One-sixth as sweet as table sugar, it is added to food as a slightly sweet source of carbohydrate. Milk turns sour when bacteria converts lactose to lactic acid.

Lecithin

Function: Emulsifier, antioxidant.
Used in: Baked goods, margarine, chocolate, ice cream.

A common constituent of animal and plant tissues, lecithin is a source of the nutrient choline. It keeps oil and water from separating, retards rancidity, reduces spattering in a frying pan, and leads to fluffier cakes. Major sources are egg yolk and soybeans.

Mannitol

Function: Sweetener, other uses.
Used in: Chewing gum, low-calorie foods.

Not quite as sweet as sugar and poorly absorbed by the body, mannitol contributes only half as many calories as sugar. Used as the "dust" on chewing gum, it prevents gum from absorbing moisture and becoming sticky. Safe.

Mono- and Diglycerides

Function: Emulsifiers.
Used in: Baked goods, margarine, candy, peanut butter.

Makes bread softer and prevents staling, improves the stability of margarine, makes caramels less sticky, and prevents the oil in peanut butter from separating. Mono- and diglycerides are safe, though most foods they are used in are high in refined flour, sugar, or fat.

Polysorbate 60

Function: Emulsifier.
Used in: Baked goods, frozen desserts, imitation dairy products.

Polysorbate 60 is short for polyoxyethylene-(20)-sorbitan monostearate. It and its close relatives, Polysorbate 65 and 80, are synthetic but appear to be safe. These chemicals work the same way as mono- and diglycerides, but smaller amounts are needed. They keep baked goods from going stale, keep dill oil dissolved in bottled dill pickles, help coffee whiteners dissolve in coffee, and prevent oil from separating out of artificial whipped cream.

Sodium Benzoate

Used in: Fruit juice, carbonated drinks, pickles, preserves.

Manufacturers have used sodium benzoate for over 70 years to prevent the growth of micro-organisms in acidic foods.

Sodium Carboxymethylcellulose (CMC)

Function: Thickening and stabilizing agent, prevents sugar from crystallizing.

Used in: Ice cream, beer, pie fillings, icings, diet foods, candy.

CMC is made by reacting cellulose with a derivative of acetic acid. Studies indicate it is safe.

Sorbic Acid, Potassium Sorbate

Function: Prevents growth of mold and bacteria.
Used in: Cheese, syrup, jelly, cake, wine, dry fruits.

Sorbic acid occurs naturally in the berries of the mountain ash. Sorbate may be a safe replacement for sodium nitrite in bacon.

Sorbitan Monostearate

Function: Emulsifier.
Used in: Cakes, candy, frozen pudding, icing.

Like mono- and diglycerides and poly-sorbates, this additive keeps oil and water mixed together. In chocolate candy, it prevents the discoloration that normally occurs when the candy is warmed up and then cooled down.

Sorbitol

Function: Sweetener, thickening agent, maintains moisture.
Used in: Dietetic drinks and foods, candy, shredded coconut, chewing gum.

Sorbitol occurs naturally in fruits and berries and is a close relative of the sugars. It is half as sweet as sugar. It is used in non-cariogenic chewing gum because oral bacteria do not metabolize it well. Large amounts of sorbitol (2 oz. for adults) have a laxative effect, but otherwise it is safe. Diabetics use sorbitol because it is absorbed slowly and does not cause blood sugar to increase rapidly.

Starch, Modified Starch

Function: Thickening agent.
Used in: Soup, gravy, baby foods.

Starch, the major component of flour, potatoes, and corn, is used as a thickening agent. However, it does not dissolve in cold water. Chemists have solved this problem by reacting starch with various chemicals. These modified starches are added to some foods to improve their consistency and keep the solids suspended. Starch and modified starches make foods look thicker and richer than they really are.

Vanillin, Ethyl Vanillin

Function: Substitute for vanilla.
Used in: Ice cream, baked goods, beverages, chocolate, candy, gelatin desserts.

CAUTION

These additives may be unsafe, are poorly tested, or are used in foods we eat too much of:

Artificial Flavoring

Function: Flavoring.
Used in: Soda pop, candy, breakfast cereals, gelatin desserts, many others.

Hundreds of chemicals are used to mimic natural flavors; many may be used in a single flavoring, such as for cherry soda pop. Most flavoring chemicals also occur in nature and are probably safe, but they may cause hyperactivity in some sensitive children. Artificial flavorings are used almost exclusively in junk foods; their use indicates that the real thing (usually fruit) has been left out.

Butylated Hydroxyanisole (BHA)

Function: Antioxidant.
Used in: Cereals, chewing gum, potato chips, vegetable oil.

BHA retards rancidity in fats, oils, and oil-containing foods. It appears to be safer than BHT (see additives to avoid) but needs to be better tested. This synthetic chemical can often be replaced by safer chemicals.

Corn Syrup

Function: Sweetener, thickener.
Used in: Candy, toppings, syrups, snack foods, imitation dairy foods.

Corn syrup is a sweet, thick liquid made by treating corn starch with acids or enzymes. It may be dried and used as corn syrup solids in coffee whiteners and other dry products. Corn syrup contains no nutritional value other than calcium; it promotes tooth decay and is used mainly in low-nutrition foods.

Dextrose (Glucose, Corn Sugar)

Function: Sweetener, coloring agent.
Used in: Bread, caramel, soda pop, cookies, many other foods.

Dextrose is an important chemical in every living organism. A sugar, it is a source of sweetness in fruits and honey. Added to foods as sweetener, it represents empty calories and contributes to tooth decay. Dextrose turns brown when heated and contributes to the color of bread crust and toast.

Gums: Guar, Locust Bean, Arabic, Furcelleran, Ghatti, Karaya, and Tragacanth

Function: Thickening agents, stabilizers.
Used in: Beverages, ice cream, frozen pudding, salad dressing, dough, cottage cheese, candy, drink mixes.

Gums derive from natural sources (bushes, trees, or seaweed) and are poorly tested. They are used to thicken foods, prevent sugar crystals from forming in candy, stabilize beer foam (arabic), form a gel in pudding (furcelleran), encapsulate flavor oils in powdered drink mixes, or keep oil and water mixed together in salad dressings. Tragacanth, sometimes used in McDonald's "Big Macs" and many other foods, has caused occasional but severe allergic reactions.

Heptyl Paraben

Function: Preservative.
Used in: Beer.

Heptyl paraben, short for the heptyl ester of parahydroxybenzoic acid, is used as a preservative in some beers. Studies suggest this chemical is safe, but it has not been tested in the presence of alcohol.

Hydrogenated Vegetable Oil

Function: Source of oil or fat.
Used in: Margarine, many processed foods.

Vegetable oil, usually a liquid, can be made into a semi-solid by treating with hydrogen. Unfortunately, hydrogenation converts much of the polyunsaturated oil to saturated fat. We eat too much oil and fat of all kinds, whether natural or hydrogenated. This additive needs better testing.

Monosodium Glutamate (MSG)

Function: Flavor enhancer.
Used in: Soup, seafood, cheese, sauces, stews, many others.

This amino acid brings out the flavor of protein-containing foods. Large amounts of MSG fed to infant mice destroyed nerve cells in the brain. Public pressure forced baby food companies to stop using MSG. MSG also causes "Chinese Restaurant Syndrome" (burning sensation in the back of the neck and forearms, tightness of the chest, and headache). Symptoms appear from 20 to 30 minutes after eating and last about an hour.

Phosphoric Acid, Phosphates

Function: Acidulant, chelating agent, buffer, emulsifier, nutrient, discoloration inhibitor.
Used in: Baked goods, cheese, powdered foods, cured meats, soda pop, breakfast cereals, dehydrated potatoes.

Phosphoric acid acidifies and flavors cola beverages. Phosphate salts are used in hundreds of processed foods for many purposes. Calcium and iron phosphates act as mineral supplements. Sodium aluminum phosphate is a leavening agent. Calcium and ammonium phosphates serve as food for yeast in bread. Sodium acid pyrophosphate prevents discoloration in potatoes and sugar syrups. Phosphates are not toxic, but their widespread use has led to a dietary imbalance that may be causing osteoporosis.

AVOID

The following additives are unsafe in the amounts consumed or are very poorly tested.

Most artifical colorings are synthetic chemicals that do not occur in nature. Though some are safer than others, colorings are not listed by name on labels. Because colorings are used almost solely in foods of low nutritional value (candy, soda pop, gelatin desserts, etc.), you should simply avoid all of them. In addition to problems mentioned below, there is evidence that colorings may cause hyperactivity in some sensitive children. The use of coloring usually indicates that fruit or other natural ingredients have not been used.

Blue No. 1

Function: Artificial coloring.
Used in: Beverages, candy, baked goods.

Blue No. 1 is very poorly tested. There is a possible risk. Should be avoided.

Blue No. 2

Function: Artificial coloring.
Used in: Pet food, beverages, candy.

This is also poorly tested; should be avoided.

Citrus Red No. 2

Function: Artificial coloring.
Used in: Skin of some Florida oranges only.

Studies indicate that this additive causes

cancer. The dye does not seep through the orange skin into the pulp.

Green No. 3

Function: Artificial coloring.
Used in: Candy, beverages.

This needs to be better tested; avoid.

Orange B

Function: Artificial coloring.
Used in: Hot dogs.

This was used to color some hot dogs; the FDA approved it in 1966, despite shamefully poor tests. In 1978, the producer stopped making it upon discovering that it contained a cancer-causing impurity.

Red No. 3

Function: Artificial coloring.
Used in: Cherries in fruit cocktail, candy, baked goods.

This complex, synthetic dye may cause cancer.

Red No. 40

Function: Artificial coloring.
Used in: Soda pop, candy, gelatin desserts, pastry, pet food, sausage.

The most widely used coloring promotes cancer in mice; it should be avoided.

Yellow No. 5

Function: Artificial coloring.
Used in: Gelatin desserts, candy, pet food, baked goods.

The second most widely used coloring is poorly tested, with one test suggesting it might cause cancer. Some people are allergic to it as well.

Yellow No. 6

Function: Artificial coloring.
Used in: Beverages, sausage, baked goods, candy, gelatin.

Appears to be safe, but can cause occasional allergic reactions; used almost exclusively in junk foods.

Brominated Vegetable Oil (BVO)

Function: Emulsifier, clouding agent.
Used in: Soft drinks.

BVO keeps flavor oils in suspension and gives a cloudy appearance to citrus-flavored soft drinks. The residues of BVO found in body fats are cause for concern. BVO should be banned, because safer substitutes are available.

Butylated Hydroxytoluene (BHT)

Function: Antioxidant.
Used in: Cereals, chewing gum, potato chips, oils, etc.

BHT is poorly tested, is found in body fat, and causes occasional allergic reactions. BHT is unnecessary in many of the foods in which it is used; safer alternatives are available.

Caffeine

Function: Stimulant.
Used in: Coffee, tea, cocoa (natural), soft drinks (additive).

Caffeine may cause birth defects and should be avoided, especially by pregnant women. It also keeps many people from sleeping. New evidence indicates that caffine may cause Fibrocystic breast disease in some women.

Invert Sugar

Function: Sweetener.
Used in: Candy, soft drinks, many other foods.

Invert sugar, a 50-50 mixture of two sugars, dextrose and fructose, is sweeter and more soluble than sucrose (table sugar). Invert sugar forms when sucrose is split in half by an enzyme or acid. It represents "empty calories," contributes to tooth decay, and should be avoided.

Propyl Gallate

Function: Antioxidant.
Used in: Vegetable oil, meat products, potato sticks, chicken soup base, chewing gum.

Retards the spoilage of fats and oils. It is often used with BHA and BHT because of the synergistic effect these additives have in retarding rancidity. Propyl gallate has not been adequately tested, frequently is unnecessary, and should be avoided.

Quinine

Function: Flavoring.
Used in: Tonic water, quinine water, bitter lemon.

This drug can cure malaria and is used as a bitter flavoring in a few soft drinks. There is a slight chance that quinine may cause birth defects, so pregnant women should avoid quinine-containing beverages and drugs. Quinine has been very poorly tested.

Saccharin

Function: Synthetic sweetener.
Used in: "Diet" products.

Saccharin is 350 times sweeter than sugar and 10 times sweeter than cyclamate. Studies have not shown that saccharin helps people lose weight. Since 1951, tests have indicated that saccharin causes cancer. In 1977, the FDA proposed that saccharin be banned.

Salt (Sodium Chloride)

Function: Flavoring.
Used in: Most processed foods, soup, potato chips, crackers.

Salt is used liberally in many processed foods. Other additives contribute additional sodium. A diet high in sodium may cause high blood pressure, which increases the risk of heart attack and stroke. Everyone should eat less salt, avoid salty processed foods, and use salt sparingly. Enjoy other seasonings.

Sodium Nitrate, Sodium Nitrite

Function: Preservative, coloring, flavoring.
Used in: Bacon, ham, frankfurters, luncheon meats, smoked fish, corned beef.

Nitrite can lead to the formation of small amounts of potent cancer-causing chemicals (nitrosamines), particularly in fried bacon. Nitrite is tolerated in foods because it can prevent the growth of bacteria that causes botulism poisoning. Nitrite also stabilizes the red color in cured meat and gives a characteristic flavor. Companies should find safer methods of preventing botulism. Sodium nitrate is used in dry cured meat because it slowly breaks down into nitrite.

Sucrose (Sugar)

Function: Sweetener.
Used in: Table sugar, sweetened foods.

Sucrose, ordinary table sugar, occurs naturally in fruit, sugar cane, and sugar beets. Americans consume about 125 pounds of refined sugar per year. Sugar makes up about one-sixth of the average diet, but contains no vitamins, minerals, or protein. Sugar and sweetened foods may taste good and supply energy, but in most cases, people eat too much of them.

Sulfur Dioxide, Sodium Bisulfite

Function: Preservative, bleach.
Used in: Sliced fruit, wine, grape juice, dehydrated potatoes.

Sulfur dioxide (a gas) and sodium bisulfite (a powder) prevent discoloration of dried apricots, apples, and similar foods. They prevent bacterial growth in wine and other foods. These additives destroy vitamin B-1. Sodium bisulfite has caused allergic reactions in sensitive individuals such as asthmatics.

Chapter 10

MENU FOR THE LUNA DIET

Your imagination is a preview of coming attractions.

—Albert Einstein

The Luna Diet Menu is based on three things: (1) decreasing fat, calories, refined sugars, and cholesterol; (2) decreasing body fat; (3) providing "Ultimate Fitness" fuel, stamina, and energy.

After years of experimenting, I have found the following menus to be excellent nutritional choices. Several choices are given for each meal, to vary according to your own preferences. Feel free to experiment with the recommended foods discussed in Chapter 8, as long as you remember to systematically undereat and to eat only when you are hungry.

BREAKFAST

Fresh Fruit Salad

2 or 3 fresh fruits in season, sliced
2 Tbsp. raisins or currants
1 tsp. sunflower seeds
1/2 cup plain non-fat yogurt

Place fruit in small bowl. Toss with yogurt. Sprinkle with raisins and seeds. Avoid sunflower seeds if you need to lose weight.

Cantaloupe and Yogurt Delight

1/2 cantaloupe, sliced lengthwise and seeded

1/2 cup non-fat yogurt
1 tsp. bran

Fill cantaloupe half with non-fat yogurt. Sprinkle with bran and dig in.

Rolled Oats and Grapenuts

1 cup uncooked rolled oats
2-3 Tbsp. Post Grapenuts or Kellogg's Nutri-Grain Nuggets
1 tsp. Miller's Bran
1/2 cup non-fat milk

Choice of 1 of the following fruits as sweetener:

1/2 banana
1-2 Tbsp. raisins
1 fresh peach, sliced
4-6 strawberries
2-3 dried figs
2-3 prunes

Place oats in small bowl. Top with remaining ingredients. Pour on skim milk, and that's it.

Chef's Delight

2 egg whites
1/2 tomato, coarsely chopped

1/4 large bell pepper, chopped
3 large mushrooms, sliced
1/8 onion, finely grated
2 oz. skim cheese (optional)

Beat egg whites. Pour into preheated Teflon pan or other frying pan to which a small amount of vegetable oil has been added. Cook for about 1 minute, stirring constantly until egg whites begin to congeal. Stir in vegetables, cover, and simmer for about 3 minutes. Place skim cheese on top, cover again, and cook 1 or 2 minutes longer, until cheese is melted and eggs begin to puff. Do not overcook. Fold over and enjoy.

Windsprint Pancakes

1 cup Health Valley Wheat Pancake Mix or
    comparable sugarless mix.
2 egg whites beaten lightly
1-1 1/2 cups non-fat milk
Unsweetened applesauce
Fresh strawberries

Combine egg whites and non-fat milk, and mix well. Add 1 cup Health Valley Pancake Mix or reasonable facsimile, and stir until smooth. Don't overmix. Heat Teflon pan or iron skillet to medium heat. If you're using an iron skillet, make sure you use a small amount of oil in the bottom of the pan. Use about 1/4 cup of batter per pancake or as desired. Turn when top of pancake shows bubble holes. Top with unsweetened applesauce and fresh strawberries. No butter, margarine, or syrup on these pancakes! Makes 10 medium-size pancakes.

David Luna Energy Drink

4 oz. orange juice
4 oz. water (I like to dilute juice with 50 percent
    water)
1 banana or 4-6 strawberries (fresh or frozen
    unsweetened)
1 Tbsp. bran
1 tsp. brewer's yeast
6 unsalted almonds (optional)
1/8 tsp. vitamin C (powder form)

Place juice and water in blender and add remaining ingredients. You might also try using a different base, like apple juice or non-fat milk. Experiment with different combinations until you find the energy drink you like best. If you're trying to lose weight, cut the portions in half and eliminate the almonds.

LUNCH

Pita Sandwich

1 slice whole wheat pita bread
2 slices tomato
1 leaf romaine lettuce
1/4 cup alfalfa sprouts

Cut pita bread to create a pocket for sandwich and stuff with veggies.

Luna's Tuna

1 small can of tuna, packed in water
4 leaves romaine lettuce
3 fresh mushrooms, sliced in small pieces
1 tomato, sliced in small pieces
1/2 celery stalk, sliced in small pieces
1/4 cup alfalfa sprouts
Gayelord Hauser's "Spike" seasoning or lemon
    juice

Combine all vegetables except alfalfa sprouts in a small salad bowl. Top with a scoop of tuna and sprinkle with sprouts. Add Spike seasoning or lemon juice. If you prefer to make a tuna sandwich, use whole wheat or dark bread.

Spinach and Mushroom Salad

1/2 bunch fresh spinach leaves
1/2 cup fresh mushrooms, sliced
1 tomato, quartered
1 hard-boiled egg white, sliced thin
Apple cider vinegar or natural herb dressing

Wash spinach leaves thoroughly. Add mushrooms, tomato, and hard-boiled egg white. Toss together with dressing and serve at once.

Spaghetti Squash

1 medium size squash
1 cup tomato paste
1/2 tomato, chopped
1/5 bell pepper, chopped
Mozzarella skim cheese
Herbs and seasonings

Cut one medium size squash in half lengthwise. Remove seeds. Place both halves cut-side down in a pan and cook in the oven for 25 to 30 minutes at 350 degrees or until skin is tender. Upon removing from the oven, take a fork and run it through the inside of the cooked squash to fluff up the pasta-like strands. Pour one cup of tomato paste, diluted with water to consistency desired. Mix chopped tomato and bell pepper into tomato paste. Add herbs and seasonings such as basil and oregano to the squash shell mix. Top with skim cheese. Place in broiler until cheese is melted. *Molto bene! Serves 2*

DINNER

Steamed Vegetables with Baked Potato and Non-fat Yogurt

3 or more fresh vegetables, cut in large pieces
Non-fat plain yogurt
1 baked potato
1 cup cooked brown rice

Steam vegetables until just cooked but not too soft. Transfer to a bake-and-serve dish. Cut baked potato in half and top with plain non-fat yogurt (not sour cream) or a chile and tomato salsa. Serve with brown rice. One of my favorites!

Eggplant Parmesan

1 large can whole tomatoes
1 can (29 oz.) tomato sauce
1 can (6 oz.) tomato paste
3-4 bay leaves
1 medium eggplant
1 medium bell pepper
1 medium onion
2 celery stalks
1/2 lb. fresh mushrooms
4-6 oz. skim cheese

Chop pepper, onion, celery, and mushrooms and mix with tomato sauce, tomato paste, bay leaves, and whole tomatoes. Simmer sauce about 3 hours. Meanwhile, grate the cheese, and boil eggplant for about 20 to 25 minutes. When soft, cool and cut into slices. Place in baking dish, add half of the sauce and half of the grated cheese. Repeat with remaining eggplant, sauce, and top with cheese. Bake 1 hour at 350 degrees. *Variations:* Substitute zucchini or other squash for eggplant. *Serves 4*

Fresh Baked Halibut or Sole

1 fresh halibut steak or sole
1 tsp. herb seasoning
Juice of 1/2 lemon

Place halibut steak or sole in a large baking dish. Season with herb seasoning. Add lemon juice. Bake at 350 degrees for 20 minutes (or fish may be broiled with the same seasoning). Serve with a small salad.

Mom's Vegetable Soup

10 cups water
3 tomatoes, sliced
1 zucchini, sliced
1 onion, sliced
2 potatoes, sliced unpeeled
2 ears of corn
1/2 small cabbage, sliced
3 carrots, sliced unpeeled
3 celery stalks, coarsely chopped
2 tsp. sea salt or herb seasoning
2 cups cooked brown rice (optional)

Bring water to boil in large pot. Add vegetables and seasoning. Cook over low flame for 5 minutes. Add cooked rice, if desired, and serve. This is my favorite soup! *Serves 4.*

Rice Pilaf

1 1/2 cups brown rice
3 cups water
1 cube vegetable bouillon
1/2 medium onion, chopped
1/2 cup coarsely chopped or broken walnuts
    (optional)

Wash rice. Bring water and bouillon to a boil, then reduce heat and simmer with lid ajar. Note time. When rice has cooked for about 30 minutes, add onions and desired spices. Continue cooking for another 20 minutes or so, mixing in walnuts at the end. Delicious! *Serves 4*

Pasta and Salad A La Luna

Carbo loading is not just for marathoners and triathletes! Mix a fresh salad consisting of Romaine lettuce, spinach, and sliced tomatoes and carrots. Mix with a pasta of your choice. season with vinegar, lemon juice or herb dressing. No mayo!

SNACKS

Fresh Apple and Non-fat Yogurt

1 apple, unpeeled sliced in quarters
1/2 cup plain non-fat yogurt

Dip apple slices into yogurt and munch away.

Popcorn (without salt and butter!)

The Old Standby

A dish of sliced celery, carrots, jicama, and broccoli with lemon wedges for snacking during the day or as an "emergency kit."

Bran Muffins (without sugar)

Raw Vegetable Juices

Recommended juices or combinations include:

Carrot
Carrot, celery, and beet
Carrot, celery, and cucumber
Tomato, celery, and parsley
Ferraro's Salad in a Bottle

Raw vegetable juice can also be purchased at most health food stores in pint or quart containers. Do not buy it if it is more than two days old, as raw vegetable juices tend to oxidize very rapidly. If possible, buy a juicer to insure freshness.

Unsalted Wheat Crackers with Skim Cheese

Fresh Fruit

Grapesicles and Bananasicles

This one is great if you have a sweet tooth. Buy green seedless grapes, wash them thoroughly, take them off the stem, and place them on a small flat tray or dish. Place them in the freezer, and what have you got? Grapesicles!

Do the same thing with a couple of bananas. Peel the bananas, place them on a small flat tray, and pop them into the freezer. Another option is to insert an ice cream stick through the length of the bananas. Dip the bananas in skim milk and then roll them in Post Grape Nuts or Kellogg's Nutri Grain cereal. There's no refined sugar in these guys. The kids will love them, and so will you.

Roasted Chestnuts (chestnuts are low in fat)

Rice or Wheat Cakes

Chapter 11

EATING DISORDERS: FULL STOMACHS, EMPTY LIVES

Good judgment comes from experience, and experience comes from poor judgment.

—Simon Bolivar Buckner

BULIMIA

- "I feel ashamed, disgusted, isolated, and depressed."
- "It's exhausting. You're weak from throwing up, and you spend whatever energy you have left planning your next binge."
- "I've never had a meal in a restaurant with a boyfriend. I just say that I'm not hungry. I don't want the embarrassment of overeating, then having to make excuses, because I took so long in the ladies room."
- "The other night, I had a date with this nice guy from my office. I brought him home and kept him up talking until 4:30 in the morning. I knew that if he left, I would start throwing up, so I seduced him. I've done that a lot."
- "I started throwing up when I was twelve. I'll be eighteen in a couple of months. I average about four times a day."

These are all comments made by young women with the eating disorder bulimia. The most recent data from Yale University, UCLA, and the University of Pennsylvania suggests that among college women (the most susceptible group) 1 to 3 percent of women have clinically significant eating disorders.[1]

Bulimia is an eating disorder characterized by alternately binging and purging to avoid gaining weight. Women and some men gorge on large amounts of calories, then purge by self-induced vomiting, laxative abuse (up to 100 times normal dosage), fasting, enemas, diuretic abuse, and abuse of over-the-counter weight-control medications, according to Dr. Carole Edelstein, Medical Director of the UCLA Eating Disorders Clinic.

The eating episode involves the uncontrolled ingestion of large quantities of food over a short period of time. The episode is triggered by anything from emotional upsets to fierce hunger following rigid dieting. The bulimic episode, or binge eating, is usually terminated by physical discomfort such as abdominal pain. Guilt, depression, and self-disgust are often experienced following a binge.

Dr. Edelstein points out that the psychiatric implications are significant. Over 30 percent have depression requiring medication with antidepressant drugs. Recent reports in the psychiatric literature have indicated an important role for such medications in the treatment of bulimia, even where depression may not be prominent.

According to Dr. Katherine Halmi, Director of the Eating Disorders Program at New York Hospital, "Severe weight loss does not occur in bulimia. There is, however, a high association of self-induced vomiting and an abuse of laxatives and diuretics in an effort to keep weight down."

A recent article in *Environmental Nutrition* points out that, "Bulimia is commonly found among young women age 18 and older. Most are primarily from middle and upper socioeconomic classes, and most have some college education. Over half are close to their proper weight."[2]

There are several factors that need to be evaluated when looking at the causes of bulimia. A good percentage of bulimics are success-oriented young women who believe that they are judged mainly on appearance. Many are obsessed with bodily perfection. They often blame their failures on weight increases, whether or not they are actually overweight. For many young women, bulimia is a way of dealing with feelings, stress, tension, anxiety, and depression. The bulimic behavior, interestingly enough, is often learned from peer groups.

To what extent bulimics rely on the binge/purge cycle varies from person to person. In extreme cases, sufferers may binge and purge more than twenty times a day.[3] Their world is virtually confined to the kitchen and the bathroom. Others may only binge once or twice per week. Some purge their systems by vomiting; others take laxatives or diuretics or resort to rigid diets or diet pills.

The "average" binge is somewhere in the vicinity of 4,000, even 5,000 calories. However, some bulimics have been known to consume as many as 20,000 calories per binge.[5] Some bulimics have died of internal ruptures as a result of extravagant and consistent binge eating. Some spend as much as $200 per week on food.

Would a person who doesn't purge but is consistently taking diuretics and laxatives to lose weight be considered a bulimic? This may come as a surprise to many of you, but chronic abuse of diuretics and laxatives for weight-reduction purposes is a bulimic-related behavior.

People from all walks of life are affected by bulimia. The UCLA Eating Disorders Clinic has treated people such as college women, actresses, models, dancers, chefs, waitresses, dieticians, physical and occupational therapists, nurses, airline stewardesses, gymnasts, housewives, and mothers.

A large number of people currently known to be affected by bulimia are Caucasians, according to Dr. Joel Yager, Program Director of the Eating Disorders Clinic, UCLA Neuropsychiatric Institute. But Dr. Yager points out that there's also an increase in the number of blacks, orientals, and Hispanics who are being affected by bulimia. The disorder is no longer limited to middle and upper socioeconomic classes. Gays may be affected more frequently than "straights," but this has not been scientifically documented. There is no scientific data currently available on Lesbians.

Medical Complications

Medical problems associated with bulimia depend on the frequency of vomiting, the abuse of laxatives and diuretics, and the physical condition of the individual. Some of the medical complications associated with bulimia are: dental decay caused by the frequent exposure of the teeth and gums to hydrochloric acid (stomach acid); electrolyte (mineral) imbalance, particularly potassium loss, which may lead to cramping, transient paralysis, arrhythmias, and possibly cardiac arrest; irritation or inflammation of the esophagus ("food pipe"); rupture of the esophagus; dehydration; rupture of the stomach; chronic sore throat; abuse of Ipecac Syrup, an emetic, has caused problems with the heart (cardiomyopathy) and irreversible congestive failure leading to death in several patients;[6] loss of normal intestinal function due to overuse of laxatives;[7] irritable bowel syndrome and/or megacolon; chronic salivary gland swelling; chronic edema (fluid retention).

Treatment

The most effective treatment for bulimia

usually combines four approaches: (1) psycho-therapy, to teach the binger to cope differently with anxiety and fear and to work on coping with low self-esteem and a distorted perception of self; (2) self-awareness techniques such as keeping a journal of moods; (3) nutritional counseling and behavioral modification techniques to improve nutrition and have a better understanding of one's eating behaviors; and (4) medication for a percentage of patients with clinically significant bulimia.

A complete medical examination is recom-mended, particularly if the binger is a frequent vomiter or abuser of laxatives or diuretics, for all three of these purge methods may deplete the body of electrolytes, such as potassium, which are necessary for cardiac function.

Even though bulimia can be successfully treated, there is still much we don't know or understand about the disorder. It is very difficult for a person to stop binging and vomiting if he or she doesn't think there is anything wrong with it. It's also very difficult for a person to stop the binging and vomiting behavior unless that person is placed in an environment where it is impossible to binge and very uncomfortable to vomit.[8]

The New York Hospital, Westchester Division, has a hospitalization treatment program for bulimia. The length of hospitaliza-tion varies from two months to six months, depending on the severity of the illness. The patient's eating and fluid intake are monitored very carfully. All patients receive individual psychotherapy several times a week, in addition to group therapy. When appropriate, families of the patients are seen weekly in family therapy. When a patient is eating normally and is ready to leave the hospital program, arrangements are made for the patient to continue in outpatient individual psychotherapy. Dr. Halmi feels that this continued therapy is important because patients with bulimia frequently revert to binging and vomiting behavior when they are under stress.

In addition to psychotherapy, behavior modification is used to treat bulimia. While the psychotherapy addresses the underlying feelings of anger, depression, and low self-esteem, behavior-modification techniques are used to give the patient coping mechanisms to deal with the desire to binge and purge.

Through therapy, you can learn that you, not others, control your life; that the greatest mistake you can make is to try to please everyone; that you don't have to be perfect; and that there are better ways to handle disappointment, anger, and depression than abusing your body.

ANOREXIA NERVOSA

The Self-starvation Syndrome

Anorexia is an eating disorder in which primarily healthy young women and a small percentage of men undertake to starve themselves to the point of emaciation in order to control their weight. It is usually characterized by the following criteria: (1) Weight preoccupation; the anorexic is terrified of being fat, even when emaciated. There is also a distorted perception of self. Anorexics see themselves as being over-weight, when in reality they are too thin. (2) Weight loss of 15 percent or more below what would be the expected weight for height and age, in the absense of another medical cause. (3) Loss of at least three consecutive menstrual periods in women who might otherwise be regular.

A recent presentation given by Dr. Joel Yager, Program Director of the Eating Disorders Clinic at UCLA, showed a female anorexic patient who at 5 feet 11 inches had gone from 210 pounds to 76 pounds. Her goal was to get down to 40 pounds, because she felt she was "still too fat." A common characteristic of anorexic patients is a self-distorted body image. Even though many are told by family and friends that they look like a "toothpick," many continue to believe they're still too fat. An anorexic who looks like "skin and bones" can look into a mirror and still see a body that is fat. Unfortunately, the fear of becoming obese does not diminish as weight drops.

Dr. Joel Yager further points out that approximately 50 percent of female long-distance runners stop menstruating or have irregular menstrual periods. Cessation of menstruation may be an unhealthy condition in that it may contribute to osteoporosis (fragile and brittle bones). Recent studies have shown that physically active women who have stopped menstruating for at least one year have 10 to 15 percent less bone mass than regularly menstruating women who are sedentary or moderately active.[9]

Amenorrhea or cessation of menstruation may be attributed to low estrogen levels, excessive exercise, low percentage of body fat, anorexia, or a combination of these or other factors. Stopping menstruation is a danger sign that a woman should discuss with her gynecologist, even if it's due to excessive exercise.

Anorexia affects approximately one out of every 200 American women according to William Bunney, M.D., of the University of California Irvine psychiatric department. The disorder occurs primarily in females between the ages of 12 and 21 but may also occur in older women and men. The anorexic is obsessed with becoming thin. They are obsessed with food, yet they won't eat. Which brings up another point: anorexics do not have loss of appetite; they simply refuse to eat.

Causes

Anorexia is poorly understood and thought to be a symptom of mental illness. Our natural obsession with slimness has had a strong subliminal impact on many young women. I'm beginning to find it very disturbing, the increasing number of young girls (often as young as 10 years) who want advice on how to get rid of all their fat, when in reality they look fine. Many anorexics are influenced by the thin, lean models and actresses they see every day in magazines and on television. Moreover, many of the current models are leaner than models of the sixties ("Twiggy," of course, being the exception). There are two to three times more articles on slenderness and diets than there were ten years ago. Subsequently, there may be the underlying fear that if you "Don't measure up," you may not be *accepted* by your peers, the opposite sex or society. As a result, some researchers in the field of eating disorders have begun to sound the alarm on not only our societal obsession with thinness, but also on the health profession's

preoccupation with the concept of "ideal weight."[10]

Medical Problems

Some of the medical and psychological problems associated with anorexia are: severe weight loss; disrupted menstruation, (amenorrhea in women and possible impotence in men); nutritional deficiencies; temporary neuro-psychological dysfunction;[11] death, if the disorder is severe enough.[12]

Treatment

Anorexia is a serious condition that requires treatment by an experienced physician or eating disorder specialist. Most patients can generally be seen as outpatients. However, if a patient refuses to eat anything, psychiatric therapy in a hospital is usually required. If necessary, the patient may need to be fed intravenously. Even if temporarily reversed by forced feedings, anorexia can reappear.[13]

Anorexics should also *not* be encouraged to eat extremely large quantities of food at the beginning of treatment to regain lost weight. Dr. Yager *recommends increasing weight to between 2 to 4 pounds per week* recognizing that some patients start treatment so dehydrated due to laxative use, diuretics, and vomiting that they may gain water weight back much more rapidly; it's the latter that has to be carefully regulated. Eating large quantities of food during the initial phase of treatment may cause rapid shifts in fluid. Dr. Yager further points out that rapid shifts in fluid have been thought to contribute to seizures. He also adds that congestive heart failure has been reported in some patients who are on rapid weight-gain programs.

Bulimia and Anorexia Nervosa

A person can be either bulimic, anorexic, or an anorexic with bulimia. Dr. Charles Portney, a psychiatrist at St. Johns Hospital in Los Angeles explains that "the best prognosis is for someone who's only bulimic, next best is for someone who's anorexic, and the worst is for anorexics who also binge and purge."

Anorexia and bulimia can be successfully treated. If you think you have either or both, seek professional help. Don't try to cope with it alone. Discuss it with your parents and bring it to the attention of your family physician. You can also call or write to any of the treatment centers listed in Appendix C for information.

QUESTIONS AND ANSWERS ABOUT EATING DISORDERS

Q: If I have an eating disorder, could I possibly cure myself?

A: It's possible, but most bulimics and anorexics cannot overcome the problem on their own. Most will require professional help. Therefore, give yourself two or three days to see how you do. If you have the slightest problem, consult an eating disorder specialist as soon as possible.

Q: How long does it take to recover from an eating disorder?

A: Recovery from eating disorders can vary from person to person. It depends on how long the person has had the eating disorder, as well as how responsive the person is to treatment. In general, it takes at least a year of outpatient therapy for the patient to begin eating normally and feeling better about himself.

Q: How can parents help their child with an eating disorder?

A: In an article written by Kathy McCoy entitled, "Are You Obsessed with Your Weight," she gives the following advice:

Parents can help most by realizing their limited ability to change the situation and by immediately seeking professional help for their daughter or son. Parents shouldn't force an anorexic to eat or constantly watch what a bulimic consumes. The person with an eating disorder uses food as a defense mechanism. The more she has to fight over food, the more she will find ways to make the problem worse.

Parents are encouraged to seek family counseling for themselves as well as their child.

Q: Once a month, I "pig out" and throw up afterwards. Do I have an eating disorder?

A: Occasional induced vomiting does not necessarily indicate that one has an eating disorder. Rather, it is a danger signal. When the little red flags start waving, it may be indicative of pre-bulimic behavior, which is why it should not go unheeded.

CHAPTER 11 NOTES

[1] Yager, Joel, M.D., Program Director, UCLA Neuropsychiatric Institute, Eating Disorder Clinic, Los Angeles.

[2] "Bulimia—Another Eating Disorder Out of the Closet," *Environmental Nutrition Newsletter,* Vol. 5, No. 6, June 1982, pp. 1-2.

[3] Fischer, Arlene, "Help for the Woman who Stuffs and Starves Herself," *Beauty Digest,* June 1982, pp. 44-6.

[4] *Ibid.*

[5] *Ibid.*

[6] Edelstein, Carole, M.D., UCLA Eating Disorders Clinic, "Medical Complications Associated with Bulimia."

[7] "Bulimia—Another Eating Disorder Out of the Closet," *Environmental Nutrition Newsletter,* Vol. 5, No. 6, June 1982, pp. 1-2.

[8] Halmi, Katherine, *Letter of Information on Bulimia,* Printed by New York Hospital, Cornell Medical Center, Westchester Division, 1982.

[9] *Tufts University Diet and Nutrition Letter,* Vol. 4, No. 7, September 1986, p. 2.

[10] Yager, Joel, M.D., "An Overview of Bulimia," presentation given at Californial State University, Northridge, on March 15, 1983.

APPENDICES

Appendix A

WHAT MAKES A GREAT ATHLETE?

GENETICS

In most cases, a great athlete is born with a natural physical talent that consists of strength, endurance, speed, and coordination. However, if you aren't born with the "right genes," it doesn't mean that you should not try to be the very best you can be. There are many athletes who have not been gifted at birth who have gone on to become great as a result of ambition, motivation, discipline, and hard training.

PSYCHOLOGICAL FACTORS

The mental aspects of training or competing are just as important as, if not more than, sheer physical ability. Training and competing are both very cerebral phenomena—more so than most people realize. The ability to handle pressure, competition, and train intelligently are a few of the components that make up the ideal psychological profile. It's important not to choke when it counts or in key situations. It's also not enough to train hard. You have to train intelligently, otherwise you may be setting yourself up for injuries. It's necessary to adapt and make changes as you go along, particularly if you see that something is not working. The key is to listen to

your body when it talks to you, gradually peak, and execute according to plan when it counts.

MOTIVATION

You can have all the right ingredients, but if you're not motivated, forget it. To excel, the flame within you must burn very strongly. You need to be highly motivated. Duffy Daugherty was right when he said, "Some men are bigger, faster, stronger, and smarter than others—but not a single man has a corner on ambition, motivation, and desire."

Remember the ten most important two letter words in the English language:

IF IT IS TO BE, IT IS UP TO ME.

EMOTIONAL CONTENT

Most people train and compete "mechanically," that is, with no emotional content or involvement. Arnold Schwarzenegger points out that "it doesn't do any good to go through training like a blind man, to just go through the motions. Motions mean nothing. You have to realize what is happening to you. You have to want results." When an athlete is emotionally aroused either in training or competition, that athlete becomes a powerful force to contend with. The athlete becomes kinesthetically sharper and more functional, particularly if he or she is able to *generate peak performance at will.*

SOUND DIET

A Volkswagen uses regular fuel. A Ferrari needs supreme or high quality fuel. If you want quality performance, you must eat quality foods. True, you may get away with hamburgers, french fries, and Cokes for a period of time, but eventually it's going to catch up with you one way or another. Food is fuel. It can either be "life-enhancing" or "life-diminishing." If you are to become the best you can be, eat those foods that will strengthen your body, provide you with endurance, and enable you to function at a high level of energy.

APPROPRIATE TRAINING PROGRAM AND TRAINING FACILITIES

You need the right training program for specificity of exercise, good coaching (both physical and psychological), well-equipped training facilities, and in some cases the right environment.

Appendix B

WORLD, AMERICAN, AND PERSONAL FITNESS RECORDS HELD BY DAVID LUNA

In 1945, Jack Lalanne set a world record for parallel bar dips. He performed 1,000 non-consecutive dips in one hour. On December 8, 1987, I performed 1,025 parallel bar dips (non-consecutively) in one hour, thereby breaking a record that had stood for 43 years. I thought I had established a new world record until I called David Boehm in New York, the American editor for the *Guinness Book of Sports Records.* He informed me that someone in England had just performed 1,300 dips in one hour a few days prior!

Disappointed, I had to settle for the American record. On top of that, I was so sore I could hardly lift my arms above my waist. I remember taking a shower afterwards and being unable to get the shampoo in my hands up to my head. My upper body was "shot" for about five days afterwards. I also recall trying to show a few new clients some exercises with some 15-pound dumbbells the following day and being unable to lift them. They must have thought I was a wimp.

The following records are a few of the athletic endeavors I have challenged myself with over the past few years. I would, however, like to clarify one point beforehand. My reasons for including these fitness records is not to show you how proficient I am, but rather to show you what you can achieve.

1. Flag pushouts *(World Record):* Performed 23 consecutive flag pushouts at World's Gym, Venice, California, May 1987. (See Figure A-1.)
2. One-Thumb Pushups on One Arm/One Thumb *(World Record):* Performed 32 consecutive one-thumb pushups at World's Gym, Venice, California, October 29, 1987. (See Figure A-2.)
3. Chin-ups in one hour *(World Record):* 500 chin-ups (not consecutive) in one hour at World's Gym in Venice, California, on April 9, 1988.
4. Parallel Bar Dips *(American Record):* Performed 1,025 dips (not consecutive) in one hour at World's Gym, Venice, California, December 8, 1987. (See Figure A-3.)
5. Performed 7,000 consecutive bent-legged sit-ups without feet pinned in 6 hours and 20 minutes at the International Health Club in Los Angeles, April 1984.
6. Rope jumped 12,000 consecutive rotations in 1 hour and 45 minutes, Santa Monica, California, October 1982.
7. Performed 6,000 supine leg raises in 3 hours and 40 minutes in Santa Monica on June 19, 1988.
8. Named "King of the Health Clubs" by the *Los Angeles Times,* March 1982.

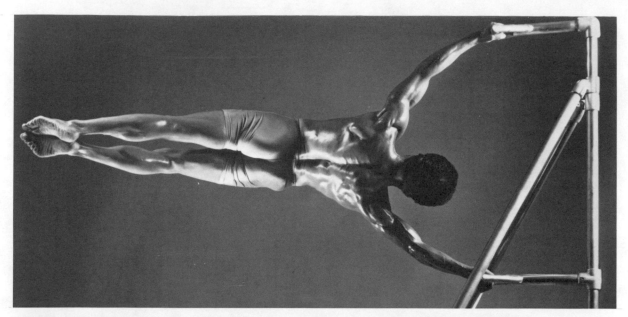

Figure A-1.

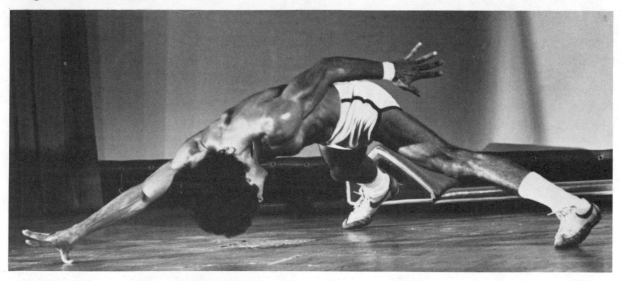

Figure A-2.

9. Ten-thousand-dollar Fitness Challenge: $10,000 to any man who can follow David Luna through a 90-minute workout. Undefeated in national and international competition.

10. Rope jumped from Santa Monica to Marina Del Rey non-stop in 6 to 8 inches of water, June 1985. Total distance traveled: 5 miles.

11. Carried twice his bodyweight (300 lbs.) one-quarter mile in Los Angeles, July 1982.

12. Performed 65 consecutive two-thumb pushups at the International Health Club, Los Angeles, August 1978.

13. Performed 20 consecutive high-bar muscle ups, International Health Club, Los Angeles, January 1977.

14. Quarter-squatted 600 lbs. three times at a bodyweight of 152 lbs. at World's Gym, Venice, California, January 1985. (See Figure A-4.)

15. Performed 2 consecutive one-armed chinups (left arm) at the International Health

Club, Los Angeles, April 1983.

16. Performed 10 consecutive calf raises while lifting 1,128 lbs. at World's Gym in Venice, California, on February 17, 1988, at a bodyweight of 154 lbs. (See Figure A-5.)

17. Performed 10 consecutive push-ups with both feet a few inches off the floor at World's Gym in Venice, California, on September 1, 1988.

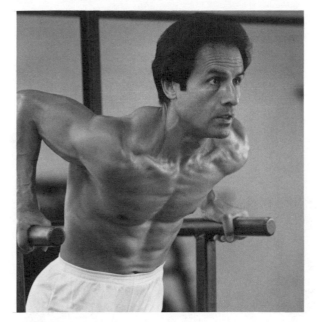

Figure A-3.

Figure A-4.

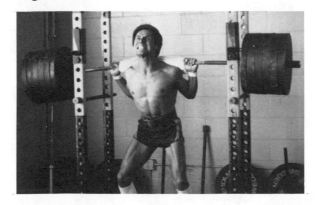

Figure A-5.

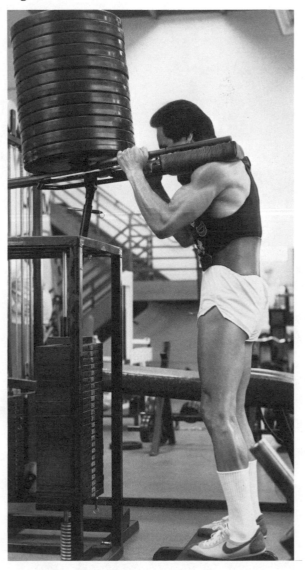

Appendix C

TREATMENT PROGRAMS

We are aware of hospital and/or clinical programs for the treatment of eating disorders at the following institutions. No doubt, many more exist. For further information, please call the Department of Psychiatry at the medical school or center nearest you, your local psychiatric association branch, or your local medical society. Many of the national self-help agencies keep current lists of professional institutions with expertise in the treatment of eating disorders.

EAST COAST

David Herzog, M.D.
Department of Psychiatry
Eating Disorders Clinic
Massachusetts General Hospital
Fruit Street
Boston, MA 02114
(617) 726-2988

Katherine Halmi, M.D.
Eating Disorders Program
New York Hospital-Cornell Medical Center
   Westchester Division
21 Bloomingdale Road
White Plains, NY 10605
(914) 682-9100

B. Timothy Walsh, M.D.
Eating Disorders Research and Treatment Program
New York State Psychiatric Institute
Columbia Presbyterian Medical Center
722 West 168th Street
New York, NY 10032
(212) 960-5752

Arnold E. Anderson, M.D.
Eating and Weight Disorders Clinic
Henry Phipps Psychiatric Clinic
Johns Hopkins Hospital
600 North Wolfe Street
Baltimore, MD 21205
(301) 955-5795

Pauline Powers, M.D.
Department of Psychiatry
University of South Florida
Tampa, FL 33612
(813) 974-2118

Mohammed Shafi, M.D.
Louisville, Kentucky
(502) 588-6941

WEST COAST

Stewart Agras, M.D. (415) 497-7107
Joellen Werne, M.D. (415) 857-0444
Department of Psychiatry
Stanford University School of Medicine
Palo Alto, CA 94305

Joel Yager, M.D. (adults) (213) 825-0173
Carole Edelstein, M.D. (adults) (213) 825-0173
Michael Strober, Ph.D. (teenagers) (213) 825-5730
Eating Disorders Clinic
UCLA Neuropsychiatric Institute
760 Westwood Plaza
Los Angeles, CA 90024

Barton Blinder, M.D.
Eating Disorders Program
Department of Psychiatry and Human Behavior
University of California Irvine
Irvine, CA 92717
(714) 831-6631

MIDWEST

Richard L. Pyle, M.D. (612) 373-8097
James Mitchell, M.D. (612) 373-8732
Department of Psychiatry University of Minnesota
P.O. Box 301
Mayo Memorial Building
420 Delaware Street SE
Minneapolis, MN 55455

Alexander Lucas, M.D.
Department of Child and Adolescent Psychiatry
Mayo Clinic
Rochester, MN 55901
(507) 282-2511

Kathleen Dixon, M.D.
Department of Psychiatry
Ohio State University

473 W. 12th Avenue
Columbus, OH 43210
(614) 421-8232

Meir Gross, M.D.
Department of Psychiatry
Cleveland Clinic Foundation
9500 Euclid Avenue
Cleveland, OH
(216) 444-5822

Sherman Feinstein, M.D. (312) 791-4181
Regina Casper, M.D. (312) 791-3878
Michael Reese Hospital and Medical Center
Lake Shore Drive and 31st Street
Chicago, IL 60616

Craig Johnson, Ph.D.
Department of Psychiatry
Northwestern University
(312) 670-4459

Troy Thompson, M.D.
University of Colorado
Denver, CO
(303) 377-4241

CANADA

Paul Garfinkel, M.D.
David Garner, Ph.D.
Department of Psychiatry
Toronto General Hospital
101 College Street
Toronto, Ontario M5G 1L7
(416) 979-2221

Appendix D

EATING DISORDERS CLINICS, NEWSLETTERS, REFERRAL, SELF-HELP, INFORMATION

American Anorexia Nervosa Association
133 Cedar Lane
Teaneck, NJ 07666
(201) 836-1800 10:00 a.m.-2:00 p.m. EST

Provides services and programs for anyone involved with Anorexia Nervosa. Interested in aiding in the education, research, cure, and prevention of this illness. Newsletter is available. Individual membership: $50.00. Newsletter only: contribution of $25.00.

A.N.A.D. (National Association of Anorexia Nervosa and Associated Disorders)
P.O. Box 271
Highland Park, IL 60035
(312) 831-3438

Offers printed material, bibliography, a poster listing symptoms, and referrals. Send a stamped self-addressed envelope.

ANRED (Anorexia Nervosa and Related Eating Disorders, Inc.)
P.O. Box 5102
Eugene, OR 97405
(503) 344-1144

Send $10.00 to ANRED in order to subscribe to a monthly newsletter. Provides information and support to individuals with eating disorders as well as their friends and families. Sponsors educational programs in schools throughout the country. Offers self-help groups for patients and their families.

B.A.S.H. (Bulimia Anorexia Self-Help)
1027 Bellevue Avenue
St. Louis, MO 63117
(314) 567-4080

Self-help for persons suffering from eating disorders. Monthly newsletter: $25.00 annual subscription.

HELP ANOREXIA, INC.
P.O. Box 2992
Culver City, CA 90231
(213) 558-0444

Offers a support group that meets twice monthly.

N.A.A.S. (National Anorexic Aid Society, Inc.)
550 S. Cleveland Avenue, Suite F
Westerville, OH 43081
(614) 896-2009

Send a check for $20.00 to become a member and receive a quarterly newsletter.

O.A. (Overeaters Anonymous)
P.O. Box 92870
Los Angeles, CA 90009
(213) 625-6252

Primarily for compulsive overeaters, but many chapters have bulimia support groups sometimes known as Vomiters Anonymous. Call or write for meetings near you.

UCLA EATING DISORDERS CLINIC
Neuropsychiatric Institute
760 Westwood Plaza
Los Angeles, CA 90024
213-825-0173

Offers comprehensive evaluation, treatment, and/or referral for individuals with anorexia nervosa and bulimia.

INDEX